INTRODUCTION TO
Exercise
SCIENCE

D1507038

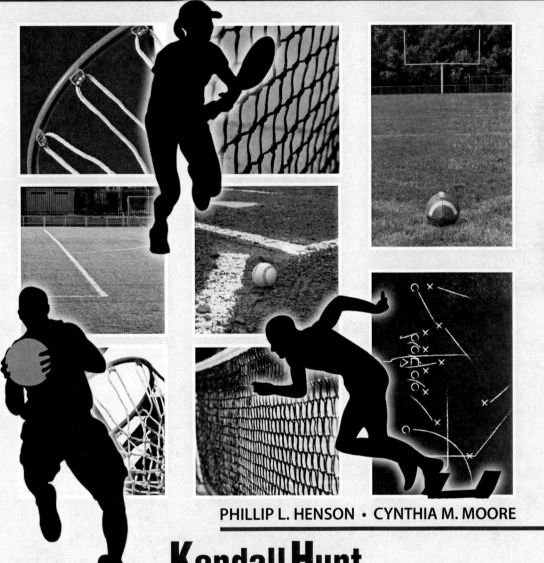

PHILLIP L. HENSON • CYNTHIA M. MOORE

Kendall Hunt
publishing company

This organization of this course is based on much of the teachings of Dr. James "Doc" Counsilman, former professor and coach at Indiana University.

I would like to dedicate this to my wife, Jane, and son, Robert, who helped organize much of the information presented in these pages. I also dedicate this project to my late parents, Burnist and Freda Henson, and to Dr. John Cooper, my mentor and friend at Indiana University. My parents and Dr. Cooper all graduated from The University of Missouri in the 1930s. Good Job, MIZZOU.

—PMH

I would like to dedicate this to my parents, Jim and Jessie Billheimer, who taught me that you can never stop learning, even when I tried. Thanks Mom and Dad.

—CMM

The authors would like to thank the following people and groups for their work and contributions to this book. Without their help, this book would not succeed.

Contributing Authors

Dr. Carrie Docherty-Steele, LAT, ATC
Dr. Dave Koceja, Ph.D.
Dr. Dave Tanner, Ph.D.
Dr. Gary Sailes, Ph.D.
Dr. Jeanne D. Johnston, Ph.D.
Dr. Joanne Klossner, LAT, ATC
Dr. John (Jack) Raglin, Ph.D.
Dr. John M. Cooper, Ph.D.
Dr. Katie Grove, LAT, ATC
Dr. Susan Simmons, Ph.D.
Indiana University School of Health, Physical Education, and Recreation
Shayla Holtkamp, MPH
Stacey Clausing, MSK

CONTENTS

UNIT III—Sport and Society

UNIT IV—Fitness and Health

UNIT V—Careers in Exercise Science

Exam Study Guides

CHAPTER I

INTRODUCTION TO EXERCISE SCIENCE

Dr. Phillip Henson
Department of Kinesiology
Indiana University

QUESTIONS FOR THOUGHT

- What makes one athlete more successful than another?

- What can coaches and scientists do to help athletes improve?

- What are the limiting factors?

- Each sport or event has inherent demands specific to that sport.

- Each individual has specific capabilities attributable to genetics and over which he or she has little control.

- An individual will have the most success in a sport or event in which his or her capabilities best meet the demands.

- Major role of coach or teacher of young athletes is to help them select their best sport or event.

FORMER EAST GERMANY AND SOVIET UNION

In the former East Germany and Soviet Union:

- Children were tested as early as 4 years old.

- They were placed in sports where they showed potential.

- They were placed in special schools.

UNITED STATES

In the United States:

- Children have well-rounded exposure instead of attempting to attain maximum potential by specializing at an early age.

- Athletes select their sport and where they want to train.

WHAT IS EXERCISE SCIENCE (SPORTS SCIENCE)

Draws information from disciplines such as:

- Biology

- Chemistry

- Physics

- Psychology

- Sociology

According to James "Doc" Counsilman, the most important areas of knowledge for a coach are:

- Physiology

- Biomechanics

- Psychology

BIOLOGICAL FOUNDATIONS

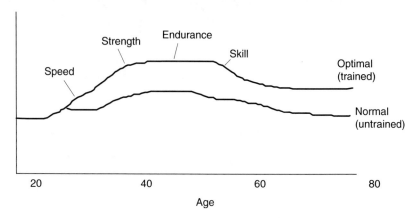

HOW THE BODY EVOLVED

- The body evolved in a far different environment than what we live in today.

- There is an inverse relationship between cultural/economic progression and physical activity.

- Therefore, planned physical activity is needed more in advanced society.

WOMEN AND ATHLETICS

- Title IX

- Scholarships

- Professional Sports

- Career Opportunities

MECHANICAL APPLICATIONS

- What is efficiency?

- What are the effects of movement in terms of . . .
  - Speed?
  - Strength?
  - Endurance?

- Do we run fast and slow the same way?

- How is movement analyzed and changed?

PSYCHOLOGICAL FOUNDATIONS

- Learning

- Cognitive

- Affective

- Motor

- Motivation

- Motor Learning – Coordination

- Personality

- Stress and Anxiety

- Knowledge

- Attitudes and Behavior

- Movement

SOCIOLOGICAL FOUNDATIONS

- What is the role of sport in society?

- What is character? Does sport build character?

- What influence does sport have on young people?

- Do sports have educational value for the participant or spectator?

CHAPTER II

THE SCIENTIFIC METHOD

THE SCIENTIFIC METHOD

- Define the problem.

- Review what others have learned.

- Form _____ (educated guess) .

- Design and perform _____.

- Make measurements and collect the _____.

- Analyze the data, draw conclusions, and make _____.

DEFINE THE PROBLEM

Ask a question.

- What are you trying to find out?

FORM HYPOTHESIS

- Make an *educated* guess to answer the question (problem). It is a statement based on what you think the results of the experiment will show.

- This is a prediction that can be tested. While it can never prove that something is always true, it can prove that it is *not* always true.

- Always based on research, be able to give reasons why you chose your hypothesis.

RESEARCH AND REVIEW WHAT OTHERS HAVE ALREADY DISCOVERED ABOUT THIS

- See what other people have already done in this area of research.

DESIGN AND PERFORM EXPERIMENTS

- An experiment is a planned way to test a hypothesis and find out the answer to the problem. Design it to test your hypothesis.

- An experiment is a way to collect data and determine the value of your independent variable, your dependent variable, and your control.

Experiment Variables

- Variables: factor that can change during an experiment.

- Independent variables: factor variable that is changed during the experiment.

- Dependent variables: factor that changes because of the independent variable.

- Controls: the one part of the experiment that must remain the same or constant throughout the experiment.

MAKING MEASUREMENTS AND COLLECTING DATA

- Develop a system of measurement: keep the system the same throughout the experiment.

- Record the data for valid results: information should be able to charted or graphed and collected in an organized format.

ANALYZE THE DATA

- What are your results?

- Perform any calculations that help you determine what the results mean — averages, percentages, totals, etc.

- Create charts, graphs, tables to represent all your data.

- Determine if results are significant.

- Look for possible sources of error — things that could make your results wrong (i.e., inaccurate measurements, contamination)

DRAW CONCLUSIONS

- Determine the answer to your hypothesis.

- Was your hypothesis supported? Why or why not?

- If you did the experiment again, what would you do differently?

- What other experiments could you do as a follow-up?

Your Results are *not* Valid If....

- They are based on opinions rather than data.

- You draw conclusions that do not logically follow the evidence.

- Your sample size is too small or is biased.

- You do not have a control.

MAKE RECOMMENDATIONS

- Communicate your findings to other scientists. Publish your findings in reputable journals of science in your area of study.

- Sharing your findings with others contributes to the growth of the body of scientific knowledge.

CHAPTER III

EXERCISE PHYSIOLOGY

Concerned with energy (capacity to perform work).

Work

A. _____ – building tissue

B. _____ – producing movement

Almost all energy originates from the _____.

TYPES OF ENERGY

Chemical

Mechanical

Heat

Light

Electrical

Nuclear

Potential

All energy is conserved (car, human body).

BASIC SYSTEMS USED IN THE BODY IN EXERCISE

- Skeletal: Provides support and range of movement

- Muscular: Produces movement (20% efficient heat 80% -- movement 20%)

- Circulatory: Transportation of O_2, CO_2, food, waste, hormones, heat

- Nervous: Controls _____ functions

- Hormonal: Controls _____ functions

- Respiratory: Provides O_2; removes CO_2

- Digestive: Breaks down food to provide energy

AEROBIC MUSCULAR ACTIVITY

- Movement performed (_____ work) when oxygen is available.

- Steady State (S.S.)

- O_2 uptake = O_2 required (_____)

- As long as S.S. is equal to or less than 50% of aerobic capacity, activity may be completely steady state.

ANAEROBIC MUSCULAR ACTIVITY

- Movement performed when _____ is limited or unavailable.

- Almost always present at the beginning of exercise.

- Muscles may function without oxygen; however, the work is accompanied by the production of _____ (L.A.).

AEROBIC AND ANAEROBIC ACTIVITY

- **Aerobic Activity**

    - May last indefinitely (limited only by amount of food, water, and O_2 available)

    - Food stored in the average person:

        1. Carbohydrates (_____ miles)

        2. Fats (_____ miles)

        3. _____ (used only in starvation conditions)

    - 1 mile = _____ KCal

- **Anaerobic Activity**

    - Has limited duration (usually limited by the buildup of _____ , whichlowers blood pH)

    - 20x more energy is produced _____ than _____ from the same amount of food

MAJOR SYSTEMS INVOLVED IN AEROBIC ACTIVITY

- **Respiratory**

    - Brings _____ into the body and absorbed into blood

    - Release _____ from blood and removes from body

- **Circulatory**

    - Transports O_2, CO_2, food, wastes, hormones, heat

    - Most O_2 and CO_2 transported by _____ which contain_____

- **Muscular**

  - Utilize O_2 and food to produce movement (20% efficient)
  - Which is usually the limiting factor in aerobic work?
    - Max VO_2 (ml O_2/kg of body wt. - Min.)

RESPIRATION

- All processes contributing to the exchange of gases
- Purpose

  1. Supply O_2
  2. Remove CO_2
  3. Maintain pH (acid-base balance)

Breathing/Ventilation

- Movement of air into and out of lungs.

- Small animals are able to _____ through the skin or through small holes in chest cavity.

- Larger animals need more surface area for _____ exchange.

- Humans have a surface area inside the lungs (alveoli) that is _____ times the surface area of the skin.

Air Passages

- Nose and Mouth

  Air is warmed and moistened

- _____

  Air is filtered

  Mucus

  Cilia

- _____ Tubes

  Branch into smaller and smaller passages

- _____

  Exchange with blood takes place

  Very thin walls surrounded by capillaries

Negative Pressure Breathing

- Accomplishes inspiration by creating a _____ pressure surrounding the lungs.

- The chest expands and causes a negative pressure inside the lungs.

- Note: Artificial respiration is a form of positive pressure breathing.

- If the chest cavity is made larger, the lungs will expand to fill this space.

Inspiration and Expiration

- **Inspiration**

  - Ribs moved _____ to increase diameter of chest

  - _____ moves downward by contracting to increase capacity

- **Expiration**

  - Normally passive (relax)

  - Forced expiration:

    A) _____ muscles (internal) contract to pull ribs downward

    B) _____ muscles contract to force diaphragm upward

Factors that Affect Lung Volume

- Age

- Height and weight

- Posture

- Absence of smoke or pollutants

- Gender

- Male 6–7 Liters

- Female 4–5 Liters

- Exercise has little effect on lung size but may increase _____ breathing capacity.

Factors that Stimulate Ventilation (Breathing)

- Increase in blood _____ detected by chemoreceptors

- Decreased arterial _____ levels

- _____ movement detected by proprioceptors

- Increase in body _____ causes increased metabolism.

- Decrease in body temperature (indirect)– _____ reflex increases metabolism

Gaseous Exchange

- _____ provides a transportation medium between the atmosphere and the body.

- External Exchange: Pulmonary ventilation or exchange in the lungs between the _____ air and the blood (98% saturated).

- Internal Exchange: Exchange between the blood and the tissue.

- Factors:

  1) Volume of blood to _____ muscles
  2) Number of open _____

Methods of Gas Exchange

- All exchange takes place by _____.

- O_2 and CO_2 move from area of _____ concentration to area of _____ concentration.

Transport of O_2 and CO_2

- **Transport of O_2**

  – Some carried in_____
  – Most carried in _____ (Hemoglobin)
  – $Hb + O_2 \longleftrightarrow HbO_2$

- **Transport of CO_2**
  - Plasma
    - $CO_2 + H_2O \longleftrightarrow H_2CO_2$
  - Hemoglobin
    - $Hb + CO_2 \longleftrightarrow HbCO_2$

The direction of each equation depends upon the relative pressures or concentrations of O_2 and CO_2 on either side of the capillary walls.

Movement of Hb and CO

- Carbon monoxide (CO)

- $Hb + CO \longrightarrow HbCO$

- Equation moves one direction only due to tight bond of HbCO

- Results in shortness of breath and eventual death.

Oxygen Inhalation in Sports

- Limited Value Because

  Blood is already 98% saturated with _____.

    – Possible Benefits of O_2
    – Breathing pure O_2 during actual exercise
    – Exercise at high altitude above 18,000 feet.
    – Psychological effects

Pain in Side (Stitch)

- Appears more often under these circumstances:

  1. Under-trained
  2. Soon after eating
  3. Downhill running
  4. Rough terrain running

Possible Causes of Side Stitch

- _____ muscle cramp

- Blood pooling in _____ or _____

- Hypoxia of _____ system

- Psychological causes

Second Wind

(Being in the "Zone")

Possible Explanation

1. Exercise begins (anaerobic).

2. Respiration falls behind.

3. Feeling of distress.

4. Respiration speeds up.

5. Feeling of relief and renewed strength.

Training Effects

- Respiration is not generally the limiting factor in _____ exercise.

- Maximal breathing may increase: Volume of Air = Tidal Volume × Breathing Rate

- _____ volume may increase in growing children.

- Chest expansion increased (stronger muscles).

- More _____ opened.

- _____ breathing is slower and deeper.

Nasal Strips

- Designed to open nasal passages to prevent snoring (ex. Breathe Rite).

- Used by Athletes to increase ventilation.

- **Questions**

  1. 90% of breathing during exercise is through the _____.

  2. Forced exhalation may increase partial pressure in _____.

CIRCULATORY

Blood

- Volume

    1. Plasma = _____

    2. Red Blood Cells (RBC) = _____

- Hematocrit = % of RBC

    1. Average in males _____

    2. Average in females _____

    **Low = _____

    **High = _____ (thick)

Red Blood Cells

- Limited _____ span (Hb is recycled)

- Production of RBCs is stimulated by low _____ levels

- Stimulate RBC Production

    1. High altitude

    2. Hemorrhage

    3. Training

Blood Boosting

- Experiments conducted in race horses

    10% increase in _____

- Benefits

    Increase in O_2 capacity

    Increase in RBCs

- Possible adverse side effects of blood boosting

    A) Old blood

    B) Polycythemia

    C) Infection

- Ethics of practice, illegal in Olympic sports

Total Blood Volume

- _____ System (1.25 L)

- _____ System (3.75 L)

    — Arteries _____

    — Capillaries _____

    — Veins _____

- Cardiac muscle

    — Contractile _____

    — Localized _____

    — Conduction _____

Blood Pressure

- _____ Pressure – Average 120 mm

  Pressure during contraction, pushes out blood

- _____ Pressure – Average 80 mm

  Pressure during relaxation, heart fills

- Good blood pressure helps blood to _____ smoothly.

Stroke Volume

- The volume of blood pumped for each _____
  of the _____

- Related to _____ of heart and _____ of contraction

- Same for left and right _____ of the heart

Starling's Law of the Heart

- The greater the heart is _____ during _____, then greater will be the quantity of blood pumped into the _____.

- The _____ attempts to pump as much blood as it receives.

- Applications

  - A _____ volume of incoming blood results in stronger, more rapid contractions.

  - A _____ volume of incoming blood results in weaker, slower contractions.

Cardiac Output

- The volume of blood pumped per unit of time (Liters per minute = L/min)

- Cardiac Output (CO) = Heart Rate (HR) × Stroke volume (SV)

- L/min = b/m × L/b (Liters/minute = beats/minute × Liters/beat)

- Average CO at rest = 5–6 L/min

- During exercise, both heart _____ and stroke _____ increase to increase cardiac output.

Examples of Cardiac Output

- Rest:

  - (SV) × (HR) = CO

  - 80 mL/b × 70 b/m = 5.6 L/m

- Exercise:

  - (SV) × (HR) = CO

  - 120 mL/b × 160 b/m = 19.2 L/m

  - This represents a 4x increase from rest to exercise.

- When HR exceeds _____ , SV begins to decline.

- When HR exceeds _____ , CO may decline.

- _____ HR is about 180.

CHAPTER IV

METABOLISM

METABOLISM

- All energy comes from the sun.

- All food comes from plants.

    Green plants manufacture food by Photosynthesis

- CO_2

- H_2O

- Chlorophyll

- Sunlight

    **Foods produced by photosynthesis
        ***Glucose (simple sugar)
        ***Cellulose (fiber)
        ***Proteins
        ***Lipids
            → All animals obtain their food directly (herbivores) or indirectly
               (carnivores) from plants
            → Sunlight + H_2O + CO_2 → O_2 + Food

OXIDATION

- Food in the presence of _____ is broken down to release energy.

- Glucose + O_2 → CO_2 + H_2O + Energy

- Oxidation → $C_6H_{12}O_6$ + $6O_2$ ←→ $6CO_2$ + $6H_2O$ + Energy

- Photosynthesis

    * _____ carry out oxidation.

    * _____ carry out photosynthesis.

ADENOSINE TRIPHOSPHATE (ATP)

- ATP is the source of energy for _____ work in the body.

- ATP is very unstable and constantly loses a _____ to form ADP with the release of energy.

- ATP → ADP + P + Energy for work

- Energy from food + ADP + P → ATP

- ATP ←→ ADP + P + Energy

LACTIC ACID SYSTEM (ANAEROBIC)

- Glucose + P + ADP → ATP + Lactic Acid

- Used for exercise of _____ intensity and moderate duration

- 10 seconds – few minutes

- Limiting factor is the build-up of lactic acid in the muscle tissue due to the lowering of pH.

- Time is required for the lactic acid to reach the liver and be reconverted to glucose.

OXYGEN SYSTEM (AEROBIC)

- Glucose or Fat + P + ADP + O2 → CO_2 + H_2O + ATP

- Used for exercise of low-moderate intensity and long duration.

- Twenty times more energy is produced aerobically than anaerobically from the same amount of _____.

- The food that does not become _____ in the lactic acid system ends up as lactic acid.

- Oxygen system can continue as long as the following are present: food, H_2O, O_2, electrolytes

- Fat is readily available for fuel, but requires more _____ to breakdown.

FOOD SOURCES

- Carbohydrates

    Preferred for moderate to _____ exercise

- Fat

    Used for _____ to moderate exercise; requires more O_2
    - 100 Kcal = 1 mile (150 lb. individual)

- Protein

    - Used only as last resort (starvation)

- Energy Sources for Exercise

    - ATP stores 1.2 Kcal

    - CP + ADP stores 3.6 Kcal

    - Carbohydrate stores 1200 Kcal (good for 12 miles)

    - Fat stores 50, 000 Kcal (good for 500 miles)

CHAPTER V

PHYSICAL WORK CAPACITY, AEROBIC TRAINING, AND MAX VO$_2$

MAXIMAL AEROBIC CAPACITY

- Definition: The highest O$_2$ uptake an individual can achieve during physical exercise breathing air at sea level.

- The more _____ an individual can consume, the more exercise he or she can sustain.

- Max VO$_2$ is expressed relative to body _____.

- mL O$_2$/Kg B.W. – min.

VALUES FOR MAXIMUM AEROBIC CAPACITY

- Average 20-year-old Female – _____

- Average 20-year-old Male – _____

- World Class Athletes:

    1. X.C. Skiers – _____

    2. Distance runners – _____

    3. Swimmers/Cyclists – _____

    4. Jim Ryan – 81

    5. Rick Wohlhutter – 82

    6. Steve Prefontaine – 84

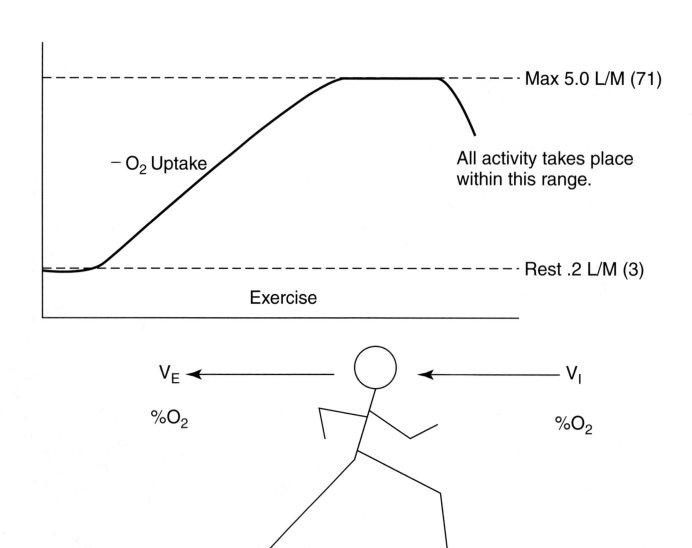

Max 5.0 L/M (71)

– O₂ Uptake

All activity takes place within this range.

Rest .2 L/M (3)

Exercise

V_E ← ← V_I

%O₂   %O₂

EXERCISE LOAD IS PROGRESSIVELY INCREASED

1. Speed

2. Grade

- Inspired

    - O$_2$ = 20.93%

    - CO$_2$ = .03%

- Expired

    - O$_2$ ~ 16%

    - CO$_2$ ~ 5%

O$_2$ INSPIRED AND EXPIRED

- O$_2$ Consumed = VE × % O$_2$I ------- VI × %O$_2$E

- Volume Inspired × Percent O$_2$ Inspired = Amount O$_2$ Inspired

- Volume Expired × Percent O$_2$ Expired = Amount O$_2$ Expired

- Difference is the amount _____

- STPD (Standard Temperature and Pressure conditions): 0°C; 760 mm Hg; 0% humidity

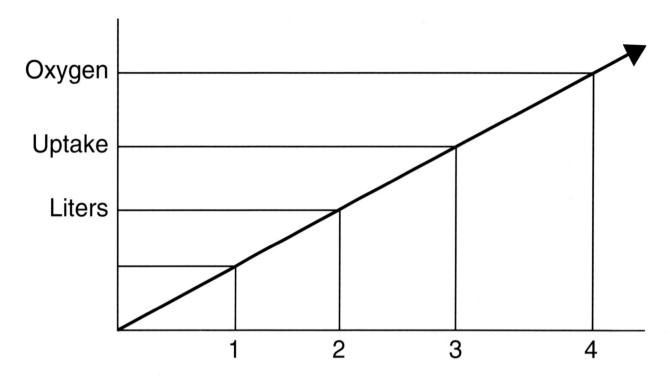

WORK LOAD

- In theory, all persons of the same weight would follow the same line.

- Fitness determines how far one can go on the line.

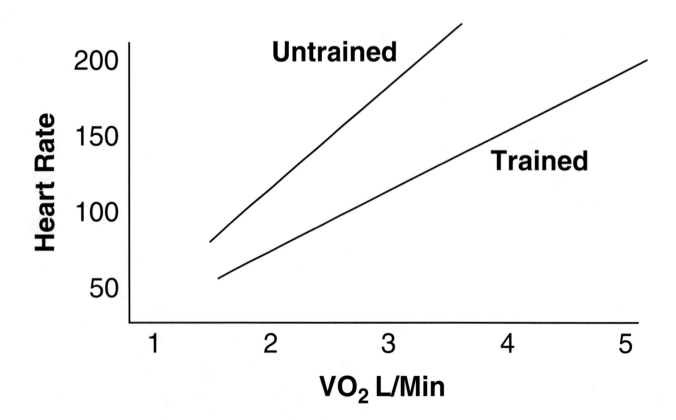

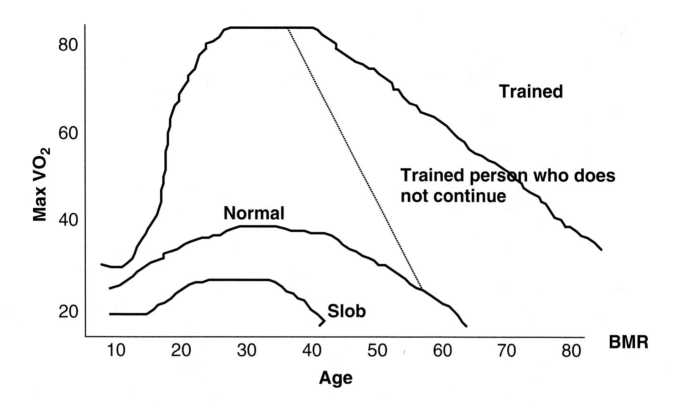

RESPIRATORY QUOTIENT

- R.Q. = CO$_2$ produced / O$_2$ consumed

- R.Q. may be used to determine the type of _____ used.

- Carbohydrate

- C$_6$H$_{12}$O$_6$ → 6CO$_2$ + 6H$_2$O

- R.Q. = 6CO$_2$ / 6O$_2$ = 6/6 = 1.00 pure carbohydrate

FAT

- $2\ C_{51}H_{98}O_6 + 145\ O_2 \rightarrow 102\ CO_2 + 98\ H_2O$

- R.Q. = $102\ CO_2$ / $145\ O_2$ .7 Pure fat

- Average R.Q. at rest = .82

- During exhaustive exercise, R.Q. may exceed 1.0, due to anaerobic work.

WHAT MAX VO_2 DOES NOT ALWAYS SHOW

- _____ – Ability to tolerate high levels of anaerobic exercise

- _____ – Ability to perform smoothly with few wasted movements

- _____ Threshold – Lactate threshold

CHAPTER VI

MUSCLE FUNCTION, BODY COMPOSITION, AND HEAT BALANCE

BODY COMPOSITION

MEN

- Average body fat –15%

- Essential fat –3%

- Athletes –5 to 12%

WOMEN

- Average body fat –20%

- Essential body fat –12%

- Athletes –12 to 20%

- Weight loss to a percentage of body fat lower than 12 can lead to:

  - Bone loss

  - Eating disorders

  - Secondary amenorrhea

MUSCLE CONTRACTIONS AND MOTOR UNITS

- Muscle _____ are responsible for all physical activity.

- Muscles only _____.

- _____ move joint in opposite direction.

- _____ are nerve and muscle fibers that work together.

- All or none.

COORDINATION

- Coordination involves the sequencing of _____.

- The number of motor units determines the strength of the contraction.

- _____ contraction not always desirable.

- A maximum contraction uses as many motor units as possible at the same time. This may not be all the motor units at one time.

- Psychology may have an effect on increasing the number of motor units contracting.

- Extreme emotional states also may have an effect on the number of motor units contracting.

INTERVENTION RATIO (NUMBER OF MUSCLE FIBERS UNDER CONTROL OF ONE NERVE)

- _____ fibers – fine motor control

- Fingers

- Eye muscles

- _____ fibers – gross movements of powerful muscles

- Legs

- Arms

- Trunk

MUSCLE FIBER TYPES

- Slow (red)

- Slow _____ activities

- High resistance to fatigue

- Fast (white)

- Fast _____ activities

- Fatigue rapidly

- _____ used to determine chemical profile

MUSCLE FIBER CHARACTERISTICS

- Fast (White)

    - _____ anaerobic activity
    - _____ capillaries and mitochondria
    - _____ fat breakdown
    - _____ Krebs cycle
    - _____ recovery
    - _____ sustained exercise
    - _____ myosin ATP

- Slow (Red)

    - _____ anaerobic activity
    - _____ capillaries and mitochondria
    - _____ fat breakdown
    - _____ Krebs cycle
    - _____ recovery
    - _____ sustained exercise
    - _____ myosin ATP

PERCENTAGE OF SLOW FIBERS

- Average population   57.7%

- Distance runners   79.0%

- Middle distance runners   61.9%

- Sprinters   43.2%

- Jumpers   34.7%

MUSCLE FIBERS

- Muscle fiber type cannot be changed.

- _____ fibers may behave as _____ fibers.

- _____ fibers may NOT behave as _____ fibers.

- Explosive tests may be used such as the vertical jump.

CHANGE IN MUSCLE SIZE

- _____ – Muscle enlargement (increase in size of each fiber)

- _____ – Decrease in size of muscle fiber

- _____ – Increased number of muscle fibers (probably does not occur)

- _____ is needed for muscle enlargement. A normal diet contains adequate _____ .

- With strength gains, _____ also hypertrophy and _____ become stronger.

- Initial strength gains for both men and women occur without hypertrophy.

- _____ is needed for large hypertrophy.

TYPES OF MUSCLE CONTRACTIONS

- Isotonic – Constant _____

- Isometric – Constant _____

- Isokinetic – Accommodating _____

- _____ – Lengthening

- _____ – Shortening

- Muscle _____ – Slight tearing of connective tissue; eccentric contractions are major causes and stretching and light exercise may help.

SPEED AND STRENGTH

- Speed is closely related to strength.

- Speed = SL × SF

- M/sec = M/st × St/sec

- For a given resistance, the greater the muscle strength, the faster the movement.

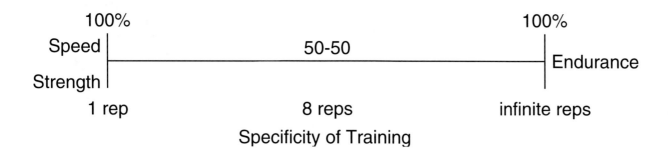

QUESTIONS...

- Can a fast fiber be strengthened with slow, powerful movements? YES or NO?

- Can endurance be increased with few, short, and intense contractions? YES or NO

PLYOMETRICS

- Eccentric contraction followed immediately by a concentric contraction

- Explosive action using fast fibers

- Stretch Reflex – Adds to strength of contraction

- Depth jumping

HEAT BALANCE

Humans as warm-blooded animals must maintain an internal body temperature of about 37° C. (~98.7°F)

Thermal death point 42°C (~107.6°F)

With types of protection humans can tolerate variations of over 132.2°C (150° F).

Temperature Control is particularly a problem during _____.

80% of energy is heat.

Transport of heat places additional stress on _____.

If the body _____ is to remain constant, heat loss must _____ heat gain.

HEAT LOSS

   1. Skin

      Most common in _____

      Aided by sweating (evaporation)

   2. Respiration _____ (in dogs)

      Panting works best if environment is below body temp.

   3. Waste Products

      Small contribution

HEAT BALANCE EQUATION

$Met \pm Cv \pm Cd \pm Rd \pm S - Ev = 0$

- _____
- _____
- _____
- _____
- _____
- _____

Evaporation 1L H_2O = 580 Kcal of heat

Sweat dripping off makes no contribution.

ACCLIMATIZATION

- Heat

      _____ sweat production (cools blood)

      _____ skin blood flow

      _____ BMR (long term)

- Cold

      _____ BMR

      _____ blood to hands and feet

Shivering

_____

Increased _____ (learned response)

CHAPTER VII

THE FEMALE IN SPORT

Dr. Dave Tanner
Indiana University Human Performance Lab
Bloomington, Indiana

FACTORS TO CONSIDER

- Physiology

- Training

- Sociology

- Special Concerns

  - Menstruation

  - Pregnancy

  - Ergogenic aids

  - The Female Athlete Triad

- **Question: Athletically, are women different from men?**

PHYSIOLOGY: ARE WOMEN DIFFERENT?

- Boys and girls are physically about equal until puberty.

    – Lean body mass is about equal up to age 13

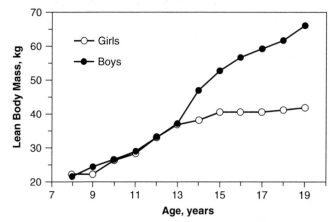

FIGURE 7–1 Changes in lean body mass with growth and aging (data from Forbes, 1972).

PHYSIOLOGY: ARE GIRLS DIFFERENT?

- Boys and girls are physically about equal until _____.

    – Motor skills are the same up to age 10–12.

- Boys practice more throwing than girls.

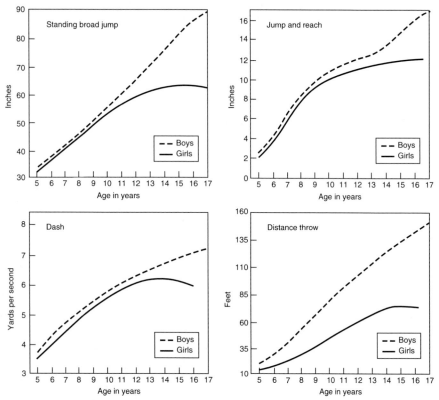

FIGURE 7–2 Performance of selected motor-skill test items for boys and girls between 5 and 16 years of age (from Espenschade & Eckert. 1974).

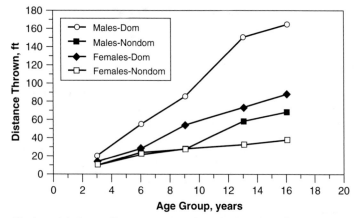

FIGURE 7–3 Softball throw for distance in males and females using the dominant and nondominant arms (from Grimditch & Sockolov, 1974, unpublished observations. University of California, Davis.

PHYSIOLOGY: WHY ARE GIRLS DIFFERENT?

- Hormones change boys to men and girls to women

  - _____

    - Increased deposition of protein, bone, etc. (LBM)

  - _____

    - Increased bone growth → growth plates close
    - Wider pelvis, breast growth, fat deposition in thighs and hips
    - More endomorphy → less body water

      Endomorphy = fatness

      Fat ≈ 10% water

PHYSIOLOGY: ARE WOMEN DIFFERENT?

Adult women and men <u>are</u> different:

- Men are taller, heavier, _____, have more muscle mass, and less fat mass

  - Men have greater mesomorphy and ectomorphy

    - Mesomorphy = muscularity
    - Ectomorphy = linearity

- Women are slower, jump lower and shorter, and throw shorter

NEUROMUSCULAR DIFFERENCES

- Men are stronger.

- But strength is equal when expressed relative to LBM.

- No difference in muscle fiber itself:

  - Muscle biopsy

  - Woman's fiber has smaller size

- Women have weaker upper body relative to lower body.

PULMONARY DIFFERENCES BETWEEN MEN AND WOMEN

- Women have _____ lung volume because of smaller size.

- Women have _____ respiratory rate.

CARDIOVASCULAR DIFFERENCES BETWEEN MEN AND WOMEN

- Women have the same max HR as men.

  – But higher HR at a given workload (to maintain cardiac output)

- The following are lower in women:

  – _____

  – _____

  – _____

  – _____

- Low hemoglobin is a potential reason for lower VO2 in women.

METABOLIC DIFFERENCES BETWEEN MEN AND WOMEN

- VO^2 is _____ lower in women

  – Highest male = 94 ml O_2/kg/min

  – Highest female = 77 ml O_2/kg/min

  – Trained females higher than average males

  – Relative VO^2 is closer when expressed as LBM, but women are still lower

    - Lower hemoglobin

    - More fat weight to carry (essential fat = 12%)

- _____ in lactate threshold (%VO_2)

- _____ in fat utilization for metabolism

ENVIRONMENTAL DIFFERENCES

- Women sweat less

  - Fewer sweat glands

- Heat acclimatization is the same as men

  - Muscles generate less heat

- Cold tolerance

  - Women have more fat for insulation

  - But less muscle to generate heat by exercise or shivering

- Altitude acclimatization is the same

PHYSIOLOGY: SUMMARY

- Almost all physiological factors for women, when expressed relative to LBM, are equal to those of men.

- Except:

  - Hemoglobin

  - Essential fat

  - Total body water

- Performance often determined by strength to weight ratio.

TRAINING: DO WOMEN RESPOND DIFFERENTLY?

- Body composition

  - Same changes as men

    - Decrease in fat mass

    - Less increase in muscle mass (less testosterone)

- Neuromuscular

  - Same changes as men but less hypertrophy

  - Increase in strength may be due to improved nerve function

- Cardiovascular

  - Same changes as men

TRAINING: SUMMARY

- Women are physically capable of performing the same training and competing in the same events (distances) as men.

- Women athletes will be more likely to approach the performance levels of men in events that do not require high levels of absolute strength, such as ultra-endurance races.

PROGRESSION OF PERFORMANCE

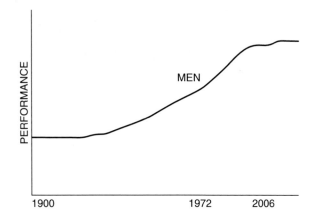

PROGRESSION OF PERFORMANCE

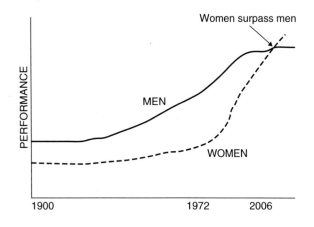

PROGRESSION OF PERFORMANCE

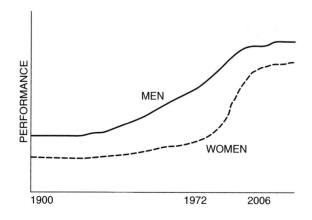

SOCIOLOGY OF WOMEN'S SPORT

- Lifestyle differences

  - Sports have been geared toward men.

  - Are sports socially acceptable behavior?

  - Women begin sedentary lifestyle earlier in life.

SOCIOLOGY: GENDER EQUITY

- Women have had fewer opportunities.

  - Men receive better coaching/funding/facilities.

  - U.S. Education Amendment, _____, 1972

    - Number of athletes proportional to number of students

    - History of expansion for women's sports

    - "Fully and effectively accommodate" interests of women students

- Results of _____

- Fewer male sports

  - Increased number of sports and athletes

  - Tremendous improvement in performance

  - Combining programs has led to fewer female coaches

SPECIAL CONCERNS: MENSTRUATION

- Menarche = onset of menstruation

  - Average age in U.S. is 12.8 years
    - Athletes = 14 years
  - Training does not delay age of menarche
  - Later age of menarche is beneficial for success
    - Taller and more linear (ectomorphy)

- Does menstruation affect performance?

  - Depends on the individual
  - World records have been set during all four phases

SPECIAL CONCERNS: PREGNANCY

- Physiological changes

  - Increased blood volume
  - Hormonal changes increase strength

- Potential concerns

  - Reduced blood flow to _____
  - _____ of fetus
    - Heat can damage fetal central nervous system
  - Low blood _____ for fetus (hypoglycemia)

- Recommended benefits of exercise

  - Improved ability to thermoregulate
  - Decrease in maternal weight gain
  - Decrease in cesareans and hospital stay
  - Lower fat mass of baby at birth

- Activities to avoid

  - Hot tubs (over-heating)

  - Competitions (high HR)

  - SCUBA diving (pressure)

  - Breath holding (resistance training)

  - Abdominal trauma

SPECIAL CONCERNS: ERGOGENIC AIDS

- Birth control pills

  - Control menstrual cycle

  - Evidence: 155 college swimmers

    - 68% of those using hormonal contraception used for non-contraceptive purposes

- Pregnancy

  - Take advantage of physiological changes

- Testosterone

  - Increase muscle mass

  - Testosterone:epitestosterone ratio < 4:1

ERGOGENIC AIDS: IS SHE "NATURAL"?

ARE THEY "NATURAL"?

WHAT IS THE "IDEAL" BODY TYPE?

THE "IDEAL" HAS CHANGED

THE FEMALE ATHLETE TRIAD

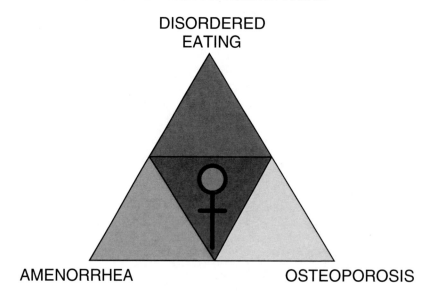

THE FEMALE ATHLETE TRIAD

DISORDERED
EATING

AMENORRHEA   OSTEOPOROSIS

EATING DISORDERS

- Anorexia nervosa and bulimia

- Prevalence can be high in athletes

  - 62% in gymnasts!

- Health consequences

  - Irreversible bone loss

  - Psychological problems, suicide

  - Cardiovascular problems

  - Reproductive dysfunction

  - Gastrointestinal disorders

  - Thermoregulatory dysfunction

  - 10-18% mortality!

MENSTRUAL DYSFUNCTION

- 2-5% in general population, but up to 66% in athletes

  - Eumenorrhea = normal menstrual function

  - Primary amenorrhea = no periods by age 16

  - Secondary amenorrhea = absence of 3-6 cycles or < 3 cycles/year after onset of menstruation

- Causes

  - Stress – caused by any of the following:

    - Training quantity or intensity

    - Low body weight or fat mass

    - Poor nutrition

    - Hormonal imbalance

- Health consequences

  - Decreased estrogen → bone loss

  - Infertility — although amenorrhea does not necessarily prevent pregnancy

- The effects are reversible

  - Except bone loss → osteoporosis

OSTEOPOROSIS

- Decreased bone density and mineral content, increased bone porosity

  - Stress fractures

- Causes

  - Reductions in _____

  - Low _____ intake

  - Inactivity

- Prevention

  - Increase calcium intake

  - Exercise, especially weight bearing

  - Estrogen replacement??

CHAPTER VIII

MOUNTAIN CLIMBING: LOW PRESSURE RESPIRATION

Dr. Dave Tanner
Indiana University Human
Performance Lab
Bloomington, Indiana

WHAT IS ALTITUDE?

- Measured as height above sea level in feet or meters

- Moderate   5,000 to 8,000 feet

- High   8,000 to 12,000 feet

- Very High   12,000 to 18,000 feet

- Extreme   > 18,000 feet

ALTITUDE OF SELECTED SITES

- Bloomington IN = 997 feet near airport

- Highest point in Indiana = 1257 feet

  – Near Richmond

- Highest point in continental U.S. = 14,494 ft

  – Mt. Whitney, California

- Highest point in North America = 20,320 ft

  – Mt. McKinley, Denali National Park, Alaska

- Highest point in the world = 29,035 ft

  – Mt. Everest, Nepal/Tibet

BAROMETRIC PRESSURE (P_{BAR})

- Measure of the weight of the column of air above you.

- Measured in millimeters of mercury (mm Hg)

  1 mm Hg = 1 Torr

  inches Hg (weather)

  millibars (altitude watches)

  1 atmosphere   = 760 mm Hg

                            = 29.92 inches Hg

                            = 1013 mbar

P~BAR~ DECREASES AS ALTITUDE INCREASES

- Sea level = 760 mm Hg = 1 atmosphere

- Bloomington IN ≈ 740 mm Hg

- Denver CO (5280 ft) ≈ 620 mm Hg

- _____ = 380 mm Hg (1/2 atmosphere)

  - Highest "livable" altitude

- 26,000 ft (death zone) ≈ 300 mm Hg

  - Supplemental oxygen

- Everest ≈ 240 mm Hg

- Space = 0 mm Hg

AIRPLANES

Pressurized to less than 8,000 feet by law.

Some people get sick anyway!

QUESTIONS:

- What percentage of the air we breathe is oxygen?

- Oxygen = _____

  $CO_2 \approx 0.03\%$, $N_2 \approx$ _____, Argon $\approx 0.9\%$

- Does this change as altitude increases?

- No! Oxygen is always _____

- Then why do we breathe more at higher altitude?

DIFFUSION GRADIENT

- Partial pressure of a gas = P_{bar} X fractional concentration of gas

- $PO_2 = P_{bar}$ X 0.2093

  - at sea level: $PO_2 \approx 160$ mm Hg

  - at 18,000 ft $PO_2 \approx 80$ mm Hg

  - on Mt. Everest $PO_2 \approx 50$ mm Hg

  - in space $PO_2 \approx 0$ mm Hg

- There must be a diffusion gradient for gas to move from lung to blood.

ANSWER TO BREATHING QUESTION

- We breathe more because P_{bar} is less.

- Therefore, partial pressure of O_2 is less.

- We have to breathe more to get enough O_2.

    i.e., the air is "thinner"

HYPOBARIC HYPOXIA

- hypo-   less than normal

- -baric   barometric pressure

- -oxia   oxygen

_____ = Less than normal oxygen resulting from less than normal barometric pressure.

- Also: Tissue hypoxia

                      Blood hypoxia (hypoxemia)

SHORT-TERM EFFECTS OF ALTITUDE

- _____ of breath during exertion
- _____ ventilation (hyperventilation)
  - stays high even after acclimatization
- _____ heart rate
  - returns to normal after acclimatization
- _____ aerobic capacity (VO_{2max})
- _____ arterial oxygen saturation (S_aO_2)
- _____ pulmonary pressure
- Changed breathing pattern at night
- Awaken frequently at _____
- Fatigue
- Increased urine output (diuresis)
- Dehydration
- Decreased blood volume

ACCLIMATIZATION TO ALTITUDE

Acclimatization = physiological adaptations that improve one's tolerance to altitude hypoxia.

- Increased _____ leads to increased RBCs
  - polycythemia
- Increased _____ density in the muscles
- Increased _____ in cells
- Increased aerobic enzymes
- Increased _____

These are all <u>good</u> adaptations.

HOW LONG DOES IT TAKE TO ADAPT?

- Depends on the individual

- Depends on the rate of ascent

- Depends on the maximum altitude

ALTITUDE TRAINING

Q: At what altitude does hypoxia begin to affect performance?

- A: Some people are affected at altitudes as low as 3000 feet!

Q: Should you train at altitude?

- A: Yes, if competition is at altitude. Otherwise, there is <u>no evidence</u> that training at altitude improves subsequent performance at sea level.

WE STILL HAVE QUESTIONS:

- What altitude is best for training?

  – Most "camps" are at 5000 to 7000 feet.

- How long should you stay at altitude?

  – At least four weeks

- When should you return to sea level?

  – Compete within 48 hours or after 7 days

EFFECTIVENESS DEPENDS ON SPORT

- May be effective for endurance athletes

  – Because of "good" adaptations

- Probably not effective for sprinters

  – Decreased intensity of training

PROPOSED TRAINING PLAN

- Sleep high – Train low

- Sleep in a hypobaric chamber or bag

SOME ALTITUDE PROBLEMS

- Decrease in physical and mental performance leads to poor judgment.

- Dehydration may lead to:

  - Hypothermia

  - Frostbite and freezing

- Anorexia (loss of appetite)

  - High altitude cachexia (HAC)

- Falls (cliffs and crevasses)

- Altitude illnesses

GOLDEN RULE I

It is OK to get altitude illness.

It is not OK to die from it.

PREDICTORS FOR ALTITUDE ILLNESSES

- No effect of age or gender

- Previous altitude illness (not always)

- Genetic predisposition (non-responders)

  – Hypoxic Ventilatory Response (HVR)

- Fitter people are more susceptible

  – Go up faster

  – Endurance athletes tend to be non-responders

ALTITUDE ILLNESSES

- Acute Mountain Sickness (AMS)

- High Altitude Pulmonary Edema (HAPE)

- High Altitude Cerebral Edema (HACE)

ACUTE MOUNTAIN SICKNESS

- Headache (primary symptom)

- Fatigue or weakness

- Loss of appetite, nausea, vomiting

- Dizziness or light-headedness

- Difficulty sleeping

- Ataxia in severe AMS

MIMIC AMS SYMPTOMS

- Dehydration

- Hypothermia

- Exhaustion

- CO poisoning

  – e.g., cooking in a tent

- Hunger

GOLDEN RULE II

If you feel unwell at altitude, it is altitude illness until proven otherwise.

GOLDEN RULE III

Never ascend with symptoms of AMS.

GOLDEN RULE IV

If you are getting worse, go down at once.

AMS TREATMENT

- Rest

- Liquids

- Descend

- Oxygen can save a life--

    . . . but it doesn't replace going down.

- Don't go up until the symptoms go down.

AMS PREVENTION

- Spend first night at intermediate altitude

- Limit exertion on first day

- Above 10,000 ft, increase < 1,500 ft/night

    – "Climb high, sleep low"

- Liquids (3 to 5 liters/day)

- High CHO diet

- Avoid alcohol, tobacco, sleeping pills

- Acclimatization

    – 24 to 48 hours

    – Depends on individual, altitude, and rate of ascent

HIGH ALTITUDE PULMONARY EDEMA

- Fluid in the lungs

- Extreme fatigue

- Breathlessness at rest, fast shallow breathing

- Cough, productive of frothy/pink sputum

- Gurgling or rattling breaths

- Chest tightness, fullness, or congestion

- Blue or gray lips or fingernails

- Drowsiness

- Usually occurs on second night after ascent.

- More frequent in young, fit climbers.

- Caused by high pulmonary blood pressure.

  - High-pressure leak or capillary damage

  - Exertion and cold exposure may contribute

- Not to be confused with:

  - High altitude cough-Bronchitis

  - Pneumonia

  - Asthma

  - Bronchitis

- Worst case result: respiratory/cardiac arrest.

Descend ASAP!!

HIGH ALTITUDE CEREBRAL EDEMA

- Confusion, change in ability to think

- Severe headache

- Ataxia

- Hallucinations

- Seizures

- Worst case result:

   – Unconsciousness, coma, death

   Descend Immediately!!

GOLDEN RULE V

Never leave someone with an altitude illness alone.

CHAPTER IX

ANAEROBIC TRAINING AND STRENGTH TRAINING

ANAEROBIC THRESHOLD

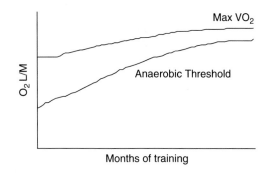

- May increase from 50% (untrained) to 90% (trained)

- 1: Max VO$_2$ = 70, A.T. = 50%, Steady State = 35

- 2: Max VO$_2$ = 60, A.T. = 90%, Steady State = 54

O$_2$ DEBT

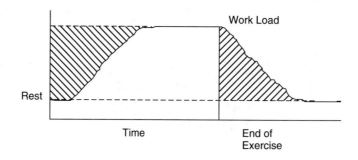

- When work load is within S.S.

- O$_2$ is needed to convert _____ to glycogen

LACTIC ACID CONVERSION

- Some lactic acid is converted to CO_2 and H_2O (elevates R.Q.)
- Oxygen Debt = Total O$_2$ needed – O$_2$ consumed

WHEN WORK LOAD EXCEEDS S.S.

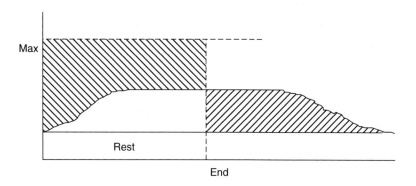

AEROBIC/ANAEROBIC COMPARISON

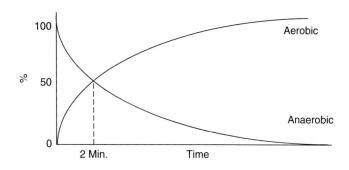

- 0–2 min = Anaerobic more important

- _____ = 50/50

- 2 – infinity = Aerobic more important

LIGHT EXERCISE

- Distance = walking

- Time = indefinitely

- All O_2 requirements met

- O_2 available in the blood

- Fat main fuel source

- No lactic acid

MODERATE EXERCISE

- Distance = marathon

- Time = as long as food is available

- Initial exercise anaerobic

- Very small lactic acid production

- Aerobic process takes over

- Lactic acid maintenance at low resting level

- Steady state

- Carbohydrate/Fat fuel source

HEAVY EXERCISE

- Distance = 3–10 Km

- Time = 10–30 minutes

- Initial lactic acid production

- Oxygen system works at peak level

- O_2 intake just meets O_2 used

- lactic acid level remains high throughout

- Absolute steady state

- More lactic acid at end

- Pure carbohydrate fuel

SEVERE EXERCISE

- Distance = 400–1500 m

- Time = few minutes

- Continuous growing O_2 debt

- Pure carbohydrate fuel

- Severe fatigue

- Continuous lactic acid production

EXTREME EXERCISE

- Distance = sprinting
- Time = a few seconds – 1 minute
- ATP – CP system and anaerobic system
- Some lactic acid buildup
- Little fuel used
- Small O_2 intake
- Moderate – severe fatigue

ALL OUT EXERCISE

- Example = weight lifting
- Time = 1–10 seconds
- Primarily ATP – CP System
- Very small lactic acid buildup
- Very small O_2 intake
- Small fatigue level

ANAEROBIC TRAINING

- Anaerobic threshold (lactate threshold):

- % of Max VO_2 at which anaerobic work begins to occur

- Untrained ~ 50–55%

- Trained ~ 80–95%

- Much of our training is designed to raise this anaerobic threshold

CHAPTER X

ERGOGENIC AIDS IN SPORTS

ANABOLIC STEROIDS AND OTHER ERGOGENIC AIDS IN SPORTS

- An **ergogenic aid** is any substance or phenomenon that is thought to elevate or improve the performance of an individual.

- Three basic questions that should be posed concerning any ergogenic aid are:

    1. _____ Does the substance do what it is supposed to do, or are the benefits merely psychological?

    2. _____ Does the substance violate any of the rules that govern the sport in which it is being used?

    3. _____ Does the potential harm of the substance outweigh the potential benefit?

WHAT ARE ANABOLIC STEROIDS?

- *Anabolic* refers to the conversion of food into living tissue or constructive metabolism.

- *Steroid* is a term used to describe certain types of hormones. Anabolic steroids, therefore, are generally thought of as synthetic hormones designed to cause increased muscle growth.

- Before puberty, most growth in the human body is controlled by _____. This process is essentially the same for boys and girls and accounts for the physical equality that is seen in boys and girls prior to puberty.

- During adolescence, sex hormones begin to play a greater role and eventually replace growth hormones as the primary cause of physical maturation.

  - In the male, this hormone is _____, which is primarily produced in the male testis.

  - Females also have very small amounts of testosterone produced by the adrenal gland, but this is relatively insignificant since it is largely overshadowed by the hormone _____.

  - Testosterone, produced in the testis of the male, stimulates the following:

    1. Increased muscle growth.

    2. Initially, increased _____ growth, but eventually also causes closure of the epiphyseal plates.

    3. The testis lowers into the scrotum and the prostate gland begins to function.

    4. The _____ changes and eventually deepens.

    5. _____ behavior increases.

    6. Beard growth begins along with other body hair.

    7. The hair line recedes, and there is an increase in potential for_____.

- Anabolic steroids are synthetic hormones, designed by pharmacologists to produce muscle growth without all the other side effects.

- They were originally designed for clinical use to treat a variety of situations, including growth problems in children, muscle maintenance in bedridden patients, and various nerve/muscle disorders.

- It was not until the late 1950s or early 1960s that athletes, coaches, and trainers began to use these drugs with the hope of increasing body size and muscular strength.

ARE ANABOLIC STEROIDS LEGAL, AND HOW WIDE SPREAD IS THEIR USE?

- Anabolic steroids have declared illegal by most sport governing bodies, including the IOC (International Olympic Committee), WADA (World Anti-Doping Agency), the IOC (International Olympic Committee), the IAAF (International Association of Athletics Federations), the NCAA (National Collegiate Athletics Association), and the NFL (National Football League).

- The exact number of athletes using anabolic steroids is unknown, but most experts agree that use is extensive. It has been reported that use may be as high as 90% in sports where body size and strength are essential ingredients

  - Professional football and baseball

  - Weight lifting

  - Certain track and field events

- NCAA and most professional sports now have established drug testing programs

  - Enforcement and penalties are much more lenient than Olympic sports

- Olympics, and sports overseen by the WADA (World Anti-Doping Agency), are very strict and the penalties more severe

  - Two-year ban for the first offense, and a lifetime ban from all Olympic sports thereafter.

- Most synthetic anabolic steroids can be detected by radioimmunoassay, or gas chromatographs

  - Look for metabolites of the various substances.

  - Until recently it was generally assumed that an athlete who had not taken steroids for five weeks or more would appear "clean" when tested.

  - Radioimmunoassay methods have now been developed with such sensitivity that they can detect usage for a period of six months or more.

  - Procedures are so sensitive that they can determine what was taken, when it was taken, and the dosage.

  - This discovery, more than any other factor, may prevent use of anabolic steroids in sports where testing is done, because two to three mandatory tests per year could effectively prevent anabolic steroid use by an individual.

DO ANABOLIC STEROIDS ENHANCE ATHLETIC PERFORMANCE?

- Much of the research on anabolic steroids is biased and conflicting.

  - Most studies using the normal dosages prescribed by a physician and untrained subject show little or no increase in muscle size and no significant increase in strength.

  - Other studies, however, using larger dosages and subjects who are trained weight lifters, show increases in both muscle size and strength.

- Unscientific observations tend to agree that athletes who begin taking anabolic steroids show remarkable increases in size and strength, provided that they have already achieved high strength levels through prior weight training and that they continued their weight training while taking the drugs.

FACTORS AFFECTED BY ANABOLIC STEROIDS

- SIZE: There is almost universal agreement that taking anabolic steroids results in increased muscle size. Disagreements center around whether this increases size is due to larger muscle fibers or is related merely to increased water retention in the tissues.

- STRENGTH: Most athletes who take anabolic steroids do so in hopes of increasing strength. It appears that athletes taking the drugs become both bigger and stronger, and this is usually reflected in improved performances in strength-dominated events.

- SPEED: Since there is a strong relationship between strength and speed, athletes who become stronger usually also increase in speed against a given resistance. Increased body size, however, may be detrimental where total body movement is required.

- ENDURANCE: There appears to be only sketchy evidence supporting increased endurance from steroids. Increased body size would definitely be detrimental for most distance runners.

- ENHANCED RECOVERY: Many athletes and physicians feel that this is the primary benefit of anabolic steroids. Athletes feel that they can train harder and more often while taking the drugs. Many athletes feel that their increased strength is a direct result of more work and only indirectly a result of the steroids.

- REDUCED INJURY: If the muscle tissue itself becomes stronger, then it will be less likely to become injured. However, muscle tissue increases in size and strength much faster than tendons, ligaments, and other connective tissue. Therefore, injuries to these structures may be more likely to occur.

- AGGRESSION: Increased aggression is a side effect of any male sex hormone (natural or synthetic), and most athletes feel they are more aggressive and determined when taking the drugs. This effect may be advantageous in competition training but can result in antisocial behavior outside the athletic or practice venue.

WHAT ARE THE SHORT-AND LONG-TERM RISK FACTORS IN USING ANABOLIC STEROIDS?

Most individuals opposed to anabolic steroids point to the risk factors when denouncing the use of the drugs.

Most side effects of steroids are time and dosage dependent and include the following:

1. Premature closure of the epiphyseal plates before growth is competed.

2. Liver damage.

3. Testicular atrophy.

4. Accelerated growth of cancer tissues.

5. Gastric ulcers.

6. Hypertension.

7. Personality changes.

8. Increased masculinity in women.

WHAT ARE THE MORAL AND ETHICAL ISSUES INVOLVING STEROID USE IN TODAY'S ATHLETIC SOCIETY?

- No athlete wants to take anabolic steroids.

  – Most athletes who choose to take steroids do so because of the tremendous pressures they place on themselves, and pressures they feel come from coaches, to improve their performances beyond what they can do with training and better technique.

  – They also feel a tremendous need to establish and maintain parity with their competitors whom they assume, rightly or wrongly, are taking the drugs as well.

- Probably the only solution to the problem is enough testing so that no athlete can take steroids without detection.

  - Then no athlete will have to take steroids to maintain parity.

- Many of the athletes felt let down by the established governing bodies of sports in the United States. For many years, most organizations, including the USOC (United States Olympic Committee), the NCAA (National Collegiate Athletic Association), and the ACSM (American College of Sports Medicine), took the position that:

  1. Steroids are illegal.

  2. Research has not proven steroids beneficial.

  3. End of discussion.

- Most of these same organizations now admit that anabolic steroids are affective and alter performances in strength and speed.

- Therefore, there is no point in discussing the matter any further.

- Proponents of steroids at the other extreme feel that the sport governing bodies should be providing physicians, physiologists, and coaches who can aid athletes in taking drugs without being detected.

  - American athletes feel that European athletes have received this type of assistance for some time and thus have a definite advantage over Americans.

- Obviously, the best path lies somewhere between these extremes.

  - We cannot bury our heads in the sand and hope that steroids will go away.

  - On the other hand, we cannot become proponents of steroids with no regard for the ethical standards of sport or the health risks of drugs.

- Continue to seek ways of achieving maximum performance without the drugs and push for strong testing programs

  - So that athletes do not feel that "everyone is taking drugs" but them.

  - Hopefully, an open-minded and enlightening approach will lead to winners based on skill and training, rather than drugs.

ADDITIONAL ERGOGENIC AIDS

- Drug taking by athletes has developed into a cat/mouse game between official testing procedures and the drugs being taken.

- As soon as a drug is outlawed and testing procedures are set up to detect it, athletes switch to a different drug or find ways to neutralize the tests.

- The following are brief summaries of drugs or procedures being used other than anabolic steroids:

  - TESTOSTERONE. Testosterone, the naturally occurring male sex hormone, has much the same effect as anabolic steroids but can be taken much closer to the testing dates without being detected. The problem is that the undesirable side effects are much more pronounced and the drug has the potential for a great deal of damage, particularly to female athletes.

  - GROWTH HORMONE. This naturally occurring hormone controls growth in children and can also produce strength gains in adults. The side effects may be much more dangerous and long-lasting than anabolic steroids. The drug reportedly costs several hundred dollars per month and is thus limited to very wealthy athletes or those who are state supported. At this point, detection procedures have not kept pace with this drug.

  - CAFFEINE. Caffeine taken in extremely large quantities can serve as a stimulant and may help the body in metabolizing fats. Athletes should be allowed to drink coffee, tea, or soft drinks, but quantities have been discovered far in excess of those normal amounts.

  - ESTROGEN (birth control pills). Large quantities of estrogens taken by females can have affects similar to those of testosterone or anabolic steroids when taken by males.

    - Although female athletes are allowed to take birth control pills, discussion has centered on limiting the amount of estrogen that may be taken by an athlete.

  - BLOOD BOOSTING. This procedure, which would primarily benefit endurance athletes, has received wide publicity but little or no testing.

    - The effects are similar to altitude training but allow exact control or manipulation of peaking. Difficulties in testing are the primary reasons that the practice has not been officially banned.

    - EPO (Erythropoietin). EPO has much the same effect as blood boosting and has now been banned by WADA. Testing requires a blood sample and results are sometimes controversial.

CHAPTER XI

NUTRITION IN SPORTS

Stacey Clausing, MSK

"Never trust a fat dietitian"?- Anonymous

WHY IS NUTRITION IMPORTANT?

"Nutrition is a valuable component that can help athletes both protect themselves and improve performance."

Bill Toomey

AN ATHLETE'S DIET

- Carbohydrate (CHO): 50–70% of total calories

    – 4 calories per gram

- Protein: 10–20% of total calories

    – 4 calories per gram

- Fat: 20–25% of total calories

    – 9 calories per gram

- Water

- Vitamins and Minerals

DIET BREAKDOWN

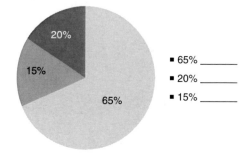

- 65% _____
- 20% _____
- 15% _____

CARBOHYDRATES (CHO)

- Primary fuel source for muscles
  - Brain and heart muscle can only use carbohydrates
- Simple vs. Complex
  - Simple
    - Processed sugars, food naturally high in sugar (fruit)
    - High glycemic index
  - Complex
    - Starches and fibers (whole grains, pasta, beans, veggies)
    - Low glycemic index
- Keeps glucose available and allows body to continue to use carbohydrate as fuel.
- Enhances body's ability to get glucose to the muscles during exercise
- Delays breakdown of glycogen in the liver until later in exercise
- Insulin levels rise after consumption, enhancing the muscle's ability to use glucose.

SOURCES OF CARBS

- Bread
- Rice
- Milk
- Yogurt
- Fruit
- Cereals
- Bagels
- Sweet potato
- Nuts
- Honey

- Fruit and vegetable juices

- Oatmeal

- Beans

- Sports drinks

PROTEIN

- Provides essential _____ to the cells

- Develops tissue to help _____ the body

- Aids in the growth of the body

- Provides enzymes, catalysts, antibodies

- Transports substances throughout the body

- Provides small amounts of energy in extreme energy deficit

- Animal Sources

  - Dairy products

  - Beans

  - Poultry

  - Red meat

  - Eggs

- Plant Sources

  - Soy products

  - Peanut butter

  - Legumes

  - Grains

FAT

- Fuel source for endurance events

  - _____ intensity, _____ duration

- Plasma membrane

- Hormone development

- Nerve cell function

"GOOD" VS. "BAD" FAT

Type of Fat	Functions for Athletes	Source of These Fats
Saturated and Trans Fat ●–●–●–●–●	Not easily broken down in the body (takes a lot of ATP)-Builds up in the arteries and contributes to heart disease	More easily broken down in the body, utilized to fuel muscles during endurance events
Mono-unsaturated fats and Polyunsaturated Fats	Butter, whole or 2% milk, marbled meats, high-fat ground beef, chicken with the skin, coconut and palm oil shortenings	Canola oil, olive oil, sesame oil, many nuts and seeds, salmon, tuna, sardines, avocados

HYDRATION

- Hydration is very important for athletes.
  - Keeps blood volume at a safe level
  - Prevents dehydration
  - Moves waste products/nutrients in and out of cells
- A _____ fluid loss can impair performance greatly.
  - 150 lb athlete = 3 lbs of sweat

WATER

- Aim for 8–10 cups of fluid/day just as a hydration base
  - 2 cups in the morning with breakfast
  - 2–3 cups ~3 hours before exercise
  - 1 cup ~10–20 min before exercise
  - ¾ cup – 1.5 cups every 15–20 min during exercise
  - 2–3 cups after exercise
  - Additional fluid at the next meal (to replace lost fluids)
    - For every lb lost during exercise, drink 2 cups of fluid

MONITORING HYDRATION

- Check your urine! If the color looks like one of these, see instructions.
  - Apple juice = drink more
  - Lemonade = you are properly hydrated

VITAMINS AND MINERALS

- Important for immune function

- Often co-factors for chemical reactions inside cells

- Important vitamins and minerals for athletes:

    - Iron – helps bind O_2 to hemoglobin

    - Calcium (phosphorus, vitamin D) – bone health, muscle contraction, nerve transmission, blood clotting

    - Vitamin C – aids in iron absorption, antioxidant, connective tissues

    - Zinc – wound healing, cell growth and repair (recover from injuries)

WATER-SOLUBLE AND FAT-SOLUBLE VITAMINS

- Fat-soluble

    - All have an "upper limit" . . . stored in fat cells and become toxic during extreme weight loss

        - Vitamin A

        - Vitamin D

        - Vitamin E

        - Vitamin K

- Water-soluble

    - No "upper limit" . . . any extra is excreted in the urine

        - Any other than the fat-soluble vitamins

SOURCES

- Fruits

  - Cherries

  - Peaches

  - Strawberries

  - Oranges

  - Pineapple

  - Kiwi

  - Grapefruit

- Vegetables

  - Broccoli

  - Tomato

  - Carrots

  - Squash

  - Potato

  - Avocado

  - Green peppers

CRAMPING

- Minerals involved in muscle contraction/catabolic work

  - Calcium, potassium, sodium

- Misconcentrations of these minerals associated with muscle cramps

  - Research unclear if hypo- or hyper-concentrations of these minerals are associated with muscle cramps.

PRE-EXERCISE

- Eat foods that digest quickly (high carbohydrate)

- Avoid new foods

- Avoid greasy, fatty, or spicy foods

- Avoid gas-producing foods (broccoli, beans)

- Allow plenty of time to digest

    - Athletes usually perform best with little to no food in their stomach

Time Before Exercise	Recommended Food/ Liquids	Pre-exercise Meal Ideas
3–4 hours	Regular-sized meal and liquid	Pasta and meat sauce, salad and low-fat dressing bread, orange juice, and water
2–3 hours	Small meal and liquids	½ turkey sandwich, banana, sports drink, and water
1–2 hours	Small snack and liquids	Cereal bar, grapes, apple juice, water
30 min. to 1 hour	Mostly liquids	Sports drink and water

- Some athletes can't digest solid foods before competition, therefore liquids are best.

    - Higher concentrated liquids take longer to digest!

- Do not try anything out of the ordinary before competition

- Remember:

    - Every person is different; athletes know their bodies best. These are just basic guidelines.

DURING EXERCISE

- Every 15–20 min you should be taking in liquids

  - Time-outs between matches or sets

- If exercise is lasting longer than an hour, you should also be taking in carbohydrates

  - A simple sports drink will be sufficient

POST-EXERCISE

- Re-hydrating

  - Again, ~ 2 cups of fluid for every lb lost

  - Monitor urine to determine hydration status

- Carbohydrates

  - Within 30 min after exercise and again 2 hours post-exercise

- Protein

  - Adding protein to your post-exercise snack aids in replacing carbohydrates and muscle recovery

POST-RECOVERY

RATIO OF 3:1 CARBS TO PROTEIN IS BEST FOR RECOVERY

- 1 cup of orange juice with 1 cup low fat yogurt

- 1 cup Gatorade and 1 Powerbar

- 1 cup apple juice and 1 peanut butter sandwich

- 1 small fast food milkshake

- 2 cups cornflakes and 1 cup low-fat milk

- 1.5 cups soymilk and 1 banana

- 1 cup of chocolate milk

  - IU study!

WEIGHT MANAGEMENT

- Weight is just a number; it shouldn't be taken too seriously

  - Fluctuations - shifts in blood volume

    - Daily

    - Monthly

    - Before / after practice

- Use to monitor change

  - Best to weigh yourself at the same time daily or weekly

- Body composition testing is useful for knowing if weight gained or lost is lean muscle or fat tissue

  - Males: 5–7%BF . . . . train best between 10–15%BF

  - Females: 12–15%BF . . . . train best between 15–20% BF

GAINING LEAN MUSCLE MASS

- Gaining muscle is not just adding protein to the diet

    - Your body needs additional energy to utilize the protein and build muscle

- Additional 1000–1500 calories per day (protein/carb/fat)

    - Gain 1–2 lbs per week

- Protein needs for lean muscle mass gain

    - Moderate Exercise : .5 –.65 gram/lb

    - Heavy Exercise: .65 – .8 gram/lb

    - Ultra Exercise/growth: .8 – 1.0 gram/lb

WEIGHT LOSS IN ATHLETES

- Any weight loss should occur in the off-season

- Weight loss should occur slowly (want to lose fat tissue)

    - Rapid weight loss

        - Water weight = dehydration

        - Lean muscle = strength loss

- Restricting diet alone is NOT the way to lose weight

    - Lack of nutrients

        - Deficiencies

        - Suppressed immune function

    - Lack of energy to maintain training regimen

- Weight loss should be no more than 2 lb per week
  - 4,000–6,000 calories per week deficit (700–1000/day)
    - Increase exercise to ~ 20 min per day
    - 1 mile of running or walking fast burns about 100 calories.
    - Decrease food intake by ~ 500 calories per day
      - Can be done pretty easily

TIPS FOR WEIGHT LOSS

- Start early- won't effect energy levels as much
- Eat small meals throughout the day; every 3–4 hours
  - Do not skip meals
- Stay hydrated – avoid high-calorie drinks
- Go easy on added fats (dressings, butter, etc)
- Try low-fat snacks (popcorn, fresh fruits and veggies)
- Tell people your plans
  - Support system
- Gradually make lifestyle changes
- Take 20 min to eat
- Know your eating style
  - Recognize stress or boredom eating
- Look at what you eat
  - Being aware makes you more conscious
- Write down what you eat
  - Easy to see where to make changes

FEMALE ATHLETE TRIAD

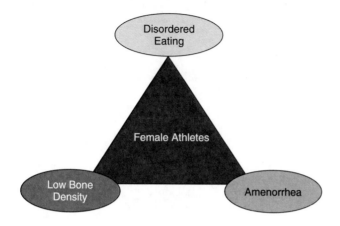

SUPPLEMENTS

- Supplementation recommended for:
    - Deficiencies
    - Stress fractures
    - Athletes withholding one or more food groups
- Iron
- Calcium (Vit. D)
- Vitamins C, E, A
- Zinc
- B vitamins
- Glucosamine/ Chondroitin

CREATINE: INCREASE MUSCLE STRENGTH AND POWER; AIDS IN RECOVERY

- Advantages

  - Taken in appropriate amounts, appears to be safe

  - Weight gain (if wanted)

  - Vegetarian athletes would benefit the most

    - Creatine found in meat sources

- Disadvantages

  - Side effects: Stomach cramping, diarrhea, dehydration

  - U.S. government does not test for safety and effectiveness of supplements. Research often done by companies selling the product

- Bottom line: Be wary of taking supplements

  - Studies show mixed results

  - Often accompanied by side effects

- Ask a professional and get his or her recommendation

  - Many supplements contain banned substances that are not reported on their labels.

JOBS OF A SPORTS DIETITIAN

- Eating on the go

- Training tables

  - Menu planning

- Athletes with special needs

  - Vegetarian athletes

  - Food allergies

  - Diabetic athletes

  - Other diseases

- Weight management

- Nutrition education

- Team meetings

- Individual consults

- Travel meal arrangements

- Healthy fast food options

- Body composition testing

- Member of support system

CHAPTER XII

INTRODUCTION TO BIOMECHANICS AND HISTORY OF BIOMECHANICS

Dr. John Cooper
Professor Emeritus
Indiana University

SAD RESULTS OF THINKING

A centipede was happy quite,

Until a frog in fun

Said, "Pray, which leg comes after which?"

This raised her mind to such a pitch,

She lay distracted in a ditch,

Not knowing how to run!

INTRODUCTORY REMARKS

1. The role of computers in our lives:

   Today almost everything you buy or have repaired involves a computer.

2. What is biomechanics?

   Bio: life and movement

   Mechanics: a synthesis of biology and mechanics in the understanding of human movement

3. *Biomechanics*: an interdisciplinary science utilizing some aspects of mathematics, physics, anatomy, physiology, and, finally, common sense.

4. Several of the world's countries have biomechanists as analysts on their Olympic coaching staffs.

5. Indiana University's biomechanics group was invited to Colorado Springs, CO, to three Olympic Festivals to analyze the actions of track and field performers.

6. High-level performers in any sport have difficulty in becoming top coaches.

   A. They have performed _____ as players and often do not know how to analyze their own performances.

   B. They often lack _____ with beginning or poor performers.

   C. They expect more than is _____ from beginning performers.

7. Every field of endeavor has a history.

8. Why would a student select this field of study?

   A. Has an interest in some human movement, example: sports

   B. Prefers to be active, not sit at a desk

   C. Believes he or she has the necessary background (or will achieve it) to be successful.

9. Seldom is there a completely new idea. A person may rearrange or substitute ideas but always must remember the origins of the initial idea. Individuals usually stand on the shoulders of others when developing ideas.

ANCIENT BIOMECHANISTS

- Hippocrates (460–370 BCE)

  – Draw conclusions only from what you perceive.

- Aristotle (384–322 BCE)

  – Studied athletes in action along with many other things

  – Started thought on this subject: subjective approach

- Archimedes (287–212 BCE)

  – Mathematics, flotation, and levers, gold or alloy

- Galen (131–201 CE)

  – Physician to the Roman gladiators

  – First to study the inside of human bodies, discovered blood flow

- Leonardo da Vinci (1455–1519 CE)

  – Greatest engineer, biologist, and artist

- Galileo (1564–1642 CE)

  – Falling bodies, tower of Pisa

- Newton (1642–1727 CE)

  – Three laws of motion

- Amar (1879–1920 CE)

  – Efficiency expert, wrote *The Human Motor*

CHAPTER XIII

BIOMECHANICS AND NEWTON'S LAWS APPLIED TO SPORTS

Dr. Phil Henson
Department of Kinesiology, Indiana University

BIOMECHANICAL FACTORS IN COACHING TRACK AND FIELD

- Biomechanics is the study of physics applied to human movement.

  - _____ motion is motion in a straight path.

  - _____ motion is motion around an axis.

  - The movement of the body Center of Gravity in running is essentially _____ movement. The movement of the arms and legs while running represents _____ motion.

  - _____ motion is motion in a curved path that describes a parabolic pathway – when athlete or object leaves the ground, it is affected by gravity

NEWTON'S LAWS OF MOTION

- Newton's First Law of Motion – Law of _____:

  - A body at rest will remain at rest unless acted upon by a force. A body in motion will continue in motion in a straight path unless acted upon by a force or friction.

- Newton's Second Law of Motion – Law of _____:

  - An object acted upon by an outside force will accelerate in direct proportion to the force and in inverse proportion to the mass of the object.

- Newton's Third Law of Motion – Law of _____:

  - For every action there is an equal and opposite reaction.

EXAMPLES OF NEWTON'S LAWS

1. Conservation of Rotary Momentum

   - Rotary Momentum – Rotary Velocity X Rotary Inertia

   - A turning body (relatively free of friction) has a constant rotary momentum. An increase or decrease in rotary inertia will result in a comparable change in turning velocity.

- Examples: figure skating, discus, high jump, pole vault

2. Acceleration – rate of change of velocity

   - _____ acceleration – speeding up

   - _____ acceleration – slowing down

   - Maximum positive acceleration takes about 6 seconds (50–70m)

- Example: A runner's body lean is a product of acceleration. At a constant velocity, body lean should only be enough to counteract air resistance (about 2° – 4°).

3. Action – Reaction

- On the ground

  – Every time one pushes against the ground, the ground reacts with an equal force.

  – In jumping and running, the greater the force, the greater the reaction.

- In the air

  – Any time a body part is moved, another body part, or the total body, must move in the opposite direction.

- Examples: high jump, hurdles

CENTER OF MASS (GRAVITY)

- The center of gravity (COG) is located about 1" above navel and 1" in front of backbone.

- Can be moved by changing body segment positions.

- Once airborne, the COG will follow a prescribed path (parabolic curve).

- Body movements may take place around the COG, but cannot change the flight path.

ROTARY MOVEMENTS MAY BE CREATED FROM THE GROUND

- Checking linear motion (javelin – long jump)

- Eccentric thrust (long jump – straddle high jump)

- Transfer of momentum (blocking)

SECONDARY AXES OF ROTATION (AXIS NOT THROUGH COG)

- Athlete may use secondary axis to affect total body rotation

    – i.e., long jump hitch-kick

MOMENT OF INERTIA

- An athlete who brings arms and legs close to the COG will spin _____.

- A long body will rotate _____.

PATH OF FLIGHT

Factors:

1. _____ of release (most important)

2. _____ of release

   – shot 41° – 42°

   – discus and javelin 3° – 40°

   – long jump 22° – 22°

3. _____ of release (determined by size and technique of the athlete)

WHAT INSTRUMENTS ARE USED TO STUDY BIOMECHANICS?

- Human eye

- Timing devices

- Optical devices (film and video)

- Electromyography

- Force plates

- Computers

LAWS AND PHYSICAL ACTION PRINCIPLES USED IN BASKETBALL

- Attenuation

- Momentum

- Quickness, speed, and velocity

- Acceleration

- Angle of incidence and inclination

- Braking force

- Center of gravity

- Elasticity

- Curvilinear

- Fatigue

- Follow through

- Impulse

- Plyometrics

- Reaction time

- Vertical jump

SELECTED TERMS

- *Attenuation* -- reduction or absorption of force

- *Acceleration* -- time rate of change in velocity

- *Center of gravity* -- that point at which the body will balance

- *Friction* -- the rubbing together of two bodies

- *Impulse* -- product of force and duration of the application of this force

- *Momentum* -- force with which a body moves; a product of a body mass and its velocity

- *Quickness* -- initial fast speed, quick to start, turn and go in any direction

- *Speed* -- a scale or quantity denoting distance per unit of time such as meters per second

- *Velocity* -- a vector quantity, denoted speed in a given direction

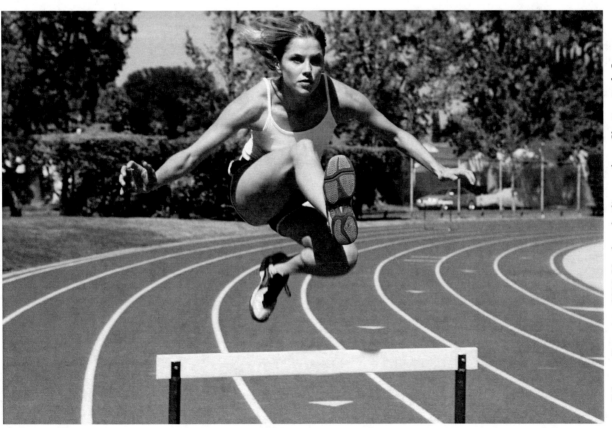

WHEN SHOULD ONE BEGIN TO PLAY A SPORT?

It depends on the desire and interest

- Tiger Woods started to play golf at the age of three. Certainly, one should not wait until retirement to try to play golf.

- It has been stated by some swimming instructors that children should be introduced to a water environment at 6 months of age or sooner. There are many adults who do not swim, so in an emergency, they flounder.

WHY IS IT HARD TO ANALYZE A TEAM?

1. Each performer is somewhat an individualist.

2. Some performers are on a team because they are more team oriented, but less talented as individuals.

3. Other team's players may disrupt moves of best opposing players.

   It is hard to study offense without considering the defense.

4. This is why most biomechanists study individual sports.

JOBS IN THE FIELD

- Work with the elderly

- Coaching

- Teaching

- Risk Management/ergonomics

- Work in movement person oriented situations

    –Former IU student is employed in the aircraft industry using biomechanics/ergonomics degree.

CHAPTER XIV

MOTOR LEARNING AND MOTOR CONTROL

Dr. Dave Koceja
Department of Kinesiology
Indiana University

MOTOR LEARNING

- Improvement in performance as a result of practice (retention). Difficult to measure learning, so we measure improvement in performance and/or skill.

- Motor learning came from psychology.

MOTOR LEARNING RESEARCH

- Develop models for learning motor skills

- Feedback – knowledge of results

- Motivation

- Practice schedules

- Transfer/retention

SKILL

- Skill – level of performance

  more efficient   consistency

  coordinated   correct mistakes

  accurate

  ability (general trait - born with it and can be trained)

     abilities are very specific

ABILITY

- Balance

- Endurance

- Power

- Reaction time

- Eye-hand coordination

- Speed

- Flexibility

- Depth perception

PRACTICE METHOD

- Mass vs. distributed practice

- Motivation – positive and negative

- Environment

- Feedback

CHARACTERISTICS THAT AFFECT LEARNING

- Environment
- Teacher or theorist
- Time of day
- Individual
- Memory
- Presentation method
- Size of class
- Attitude
- Readiness to learn
- Feedback
- Motivation

MOTOR CONTROL

- Mechanisms responsible for the production of movement
- Motor control came from neurophysiology

RESEARCH

- Develop models for the control of movement

    *How do we work?

- Age

- Training

HENNEMAN'S SIZE PRINCIPLE

- Muscles are composed of thousands of motor units.

Motor Units	Diameter	Speed	Number of Fibers
Large	Large	Quick	Many
Small	Small	Slow	Few

- The CNS begins with small fibers and then recruits large ones whey they are needed.

MOTOR CONTROL

- Neural plasticity – CNS can be trained

  – CNS – highly organized at every level

- Motor cortex does the programming for movement

- Muscle force:

  – Recruitment of motor units = Small then large

  – Frequency within motor units = Training plays a role

- Motor Unit = Motor neuron and all muscle fibers connected to it

CHAPTER XV

COACHING PHILOSOPHY AND LEADERSHIP

Dr. Phil Henson
Department of Kinesiology
Indiana University

CHARACTERISTICS OF A GREAT COACH

- Has complete confidence in his or her ability and in the ability of the athlete

- Passes this confidence along to the athlete

- Looked upon as a "Guru"

- Leads by _____

- Leads by _____

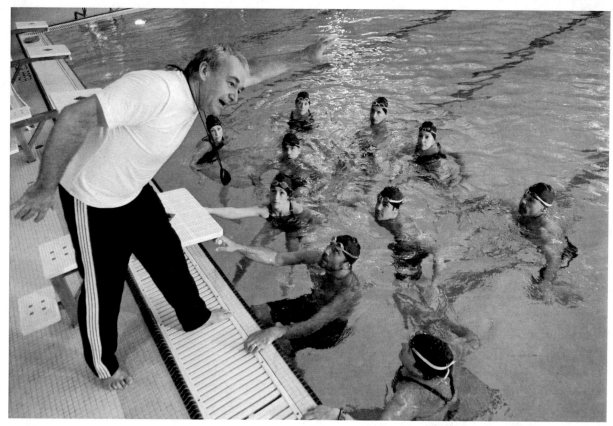

TYPES OF COACHES

- "Hard-nosed" authoritarian coach

- "Nice-guy" coach

- Intense or "Driven" coach

- "Easy-going" coach

- "Business-like" coach

CHARACTERISTICS OF THE "HARD-NOSED" AUTHORITARIAN COACH

- Believes strongly in discipline

- Usually uses punitive measures to enforce rules

- Rigid about schedules and plans

- Can be cruel and sadistic (often insulting)

- Not usually warm or personable

- Very organized and well-planned

- Doesn't like to get too close interpersonally

- Often religious and moralistic

- Often bigoted and prejudiced

- Prefers weaker people as assistant coaches

- Uses threats to motivate

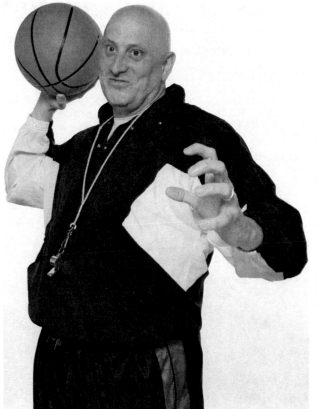

© 2010, Jupiter Images Corporation

<u>Advantages</u>

- Disciplined club

- Usually aggressive and physically punishing team

- Well-organized club

- Usually in better physical condition than other teams

- Good team spirit when winning

<u>Disadvantages</u>

- Team prone to dissension when things go badly

- Sensitive athletes unable to handle such treatment

- Coach often disliked or feared

- Team often driven and tense when unnecessary

CHARACTERISTICS OF THE "NICE-GUY" COACH

- Usually liked by a number of people

- Considerate of others

- Uses positive means to motivate athletes

- Very flexible in planning—sometimes chaotic and often experimental

<u>Advantages</u>

- Good team cohesiveness

- Athletes produce beyond what is expected of them

- Team usually relaxed

<u>Disadvantages</u>

- Coach often seen as weak

- "Con-men" not handled well

- May lose socially inhibited athletes

CHARACTERISTICS OF THE INTENSE OR "DRIVEN" COACH

- Frequently worried

- Overemphasizes or dramatizes situations

- Takes things personally

- Spends endless hours on materials

- Always has complete knowledge of the game

- Always pushing self; never satisfied with accomplishments

- Motivates players by example

<u>Advantages</u>

- Team usually "up" for a contest

- Team supported by coach when it works hard

- Coach harder worker than the athletes—proving his or her commitment

<u>Disadvantages</u>

- May frighten some athletes by being too demanding

- Possibility of team burnout before end of season or before crucial games

- May dislike athlete who appears lazy

- Depression-prone players not handled well

- Demands may be unrealistic

- Often team members ashamed of coach's emotional display

CHARACTERISTICS OF THE "EASY-GOING" COACH

- Does not seem to take things seriously

- Dislikes schedules

- Does not get rattled easily

- Gives impression that everything is under control—at times may seem lazy

<u>Advantages</u>

- Little pressure within the team

- Little griping by team about hard work

- Things more easily picked up by team and questioned more

- Greater feeling of independence from coach

<u>Disadvantages</u>

- Coach often seen as inadequate

- Coach often seen as a playboy—not interested in sports

- Team often not in top physical condition due to lack of hard work

- Pressure not handled well by team—panic may occur

- Coach often seen as uncaring

CHARACTERISTICS OF THE "BUSINESS-LIKE" COACH

- Approaches the sport in a calculating manner—well-organized

- Very logical in his or her approach

- A cool person interpersonally

- Sharp intellectually

- Major emphasis on out-thinking the opponent

- Pragmatic and preserving

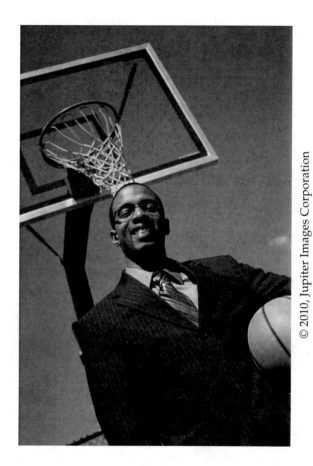

© 2010, Jupiter Images Corporation

Advantages

- Usually team up-to-date on new techniques

- Sound and organized strategy for success

- Athletes' doubts dispelled and confidence developed through intelligent organization

Disadvantages

- Feeling of unimportance in players—like pawns

- Little concern for others on team—spirit of team lacking

- Hard on disorganized athletes

- Misses athletes motivated emotionally

CHAPTER XVI

SPORT AND SOCIETY: SPORT SOCIOLOGY

Dr. Gary Sailes
Department of Kinesiology
Indiana University

SPORT SOCIOLOGY

- Scientific discipline that focuses on the interrelationship between sport and society.

- Looks at how people respond to sport in group interactions.

LEVELS OF GROUP ACTIVITY

- Play

- Games

- Sport

PLAY

- Unstructured

- Natural

- Spontaneous

- Fun

- Intrinsic rewards

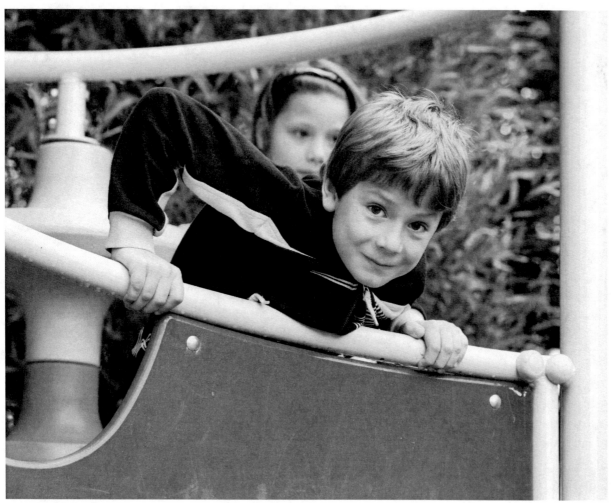

Children at play

GAMES

- More organized
- Social
- Some equipment
- Simple rules

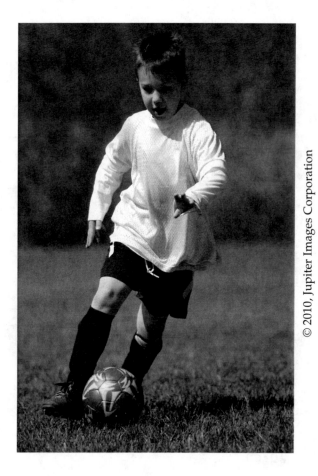

© 2010, Jupiter Images Corporation

SPORT

- Competitive

- Written rules

- Organized

- Winners and losers

- Extrinsic rewards

- Published scores

INSTITUTIONS STUDIED IN SPORT SOCIOLOGY

- Family

- History

- Socialization

- Gender

- Race

- Media

- High school sports

- College sports

- Professional sports

AMERICAN SPORT CREED

- Character building

- Develops discipline

- Competition

- Physical fitness

- Mental fitness

- Religiosity

- Nationalism

CONFLICT THEORY

- Sport brings out the worst in society.

FUNCTIONALIST THEORY

- Sports is always positive and helps to meet basic needs
- Builds cooperation

CRITICAL THEORY

- Sport a reflection of society
- Complex relationship

SPORT MIRRORS SOCIETY

- Money
- Drugs
- Race relations
  - Stereotypes
- Terminology
- Cheating
- Violence
- Gambling

GOLDEN AGE OF SPORTS

- Men: 1920

- Women: today

THE 'STATE' OF SPORTS TODAY

- Gross domestic product of sport in the United States is $324 billion.

- Is there such a thing as a "natural athlete"?

- What is "stacking"?

- Should college athletes be paid?

ARE THEY THE SAME?

- Title IX

- Gender equity

SHOULD COLLEGE SPORTS BE A "FARM SYSTEM" FOR THE PROS?

- Athletes tend to major in eligibility.

- Only 1/3 of the NFL have college degrees.

- Only 1/4 of the NBA have college degrees.

- Most MLB players never attend college.

- Average pro career is _____ years.

- Average salary following a pro career is $20,000/year.

CHAPTER XVII

SPORT PSYCHOLOGY

Dr. John (Jack) Raglin
Indiana University
Department of Kinesiology

SPORT PSYCHOLOGY

- What it is

- What it's not

Areas defined by USOC:

- Clinical

- Educational

- Research

- Interest began in _____ by _____
  at U. of Illinois

Three domains of learning:

1. _____—knowledge

2. _____—behavior

3. _____—movement

- _____—development of motor skills

- _____—mechanisms responsible for the production
  of movement

WHAT FACTORS INFLUENCE ELITE ATHLETIC PERFORMANCE?

- Exercise physiology

- Sport technology

- Environmental physiology

- Motor control

- Biomechanics

What is the role of psychology?

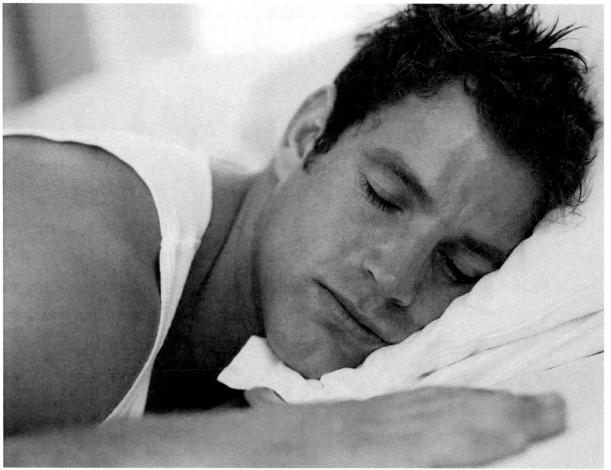

© Monkey Business Images, 2010. Used under license from Shutterstock, Inc.

Sleep

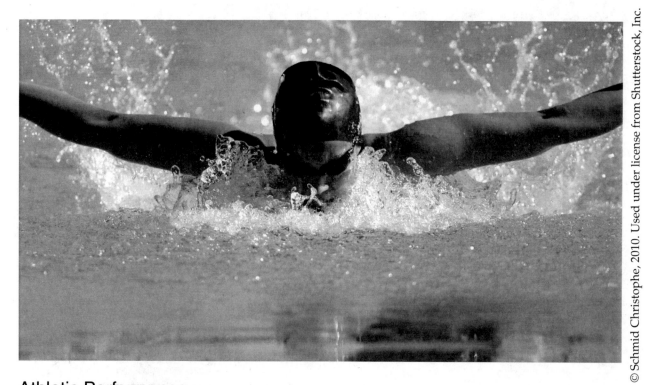

Athletic Performance

CAN SLEEP PATTERNS BE INFLUENCED?

- Relaxation

- Meditation

- Biofeedback

- Medication

Should sleep patterns be influenced?

What is the evidence?

WHO DO SPORT PSYCHOLOGISTS STUDY?

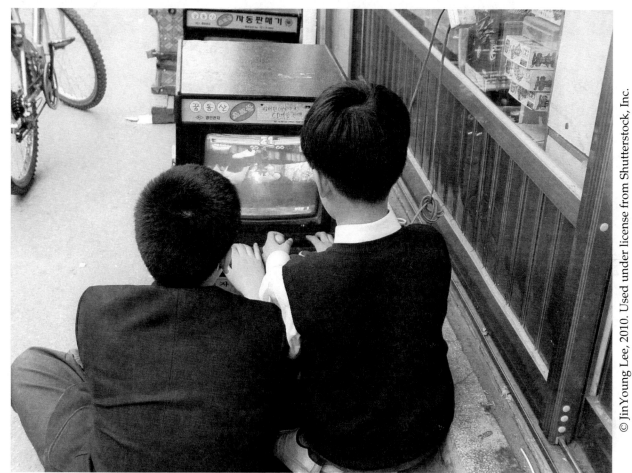

Children sitting and playing video games rather than doing physical activities.

PSYCHOLOGY AND COACHING

What is motivation?

A MODEL OF SPORT PSYCHOLOGY

Performance Psychology	anxiety depression personality	$\longrightarrow$	athletic performance (behavior)
Health Psychology	exercise or sport participation (behavior)	$\longrightarrow$	anxiety depression personality

HOW OLD IS THE FIELD OF SPORT PSYCHOLOGY?

COLEMAN ROBERTS GRIFFITH

1918: Begins study on psychological factors in football and baseball.

1923: Offers psychology and athletics course.

1925: Opens first sport psychology laboratory in the United States.

WHAT DO SPORT PSYCHOLOGISTS STUDY?

- The Stress of Competition

  - What sport psychologists say about stress and anxiety:

    - "An undesirable experience."

    - "Increased levels have a detrimental effect on performance."

    - "Responsible for athletes quitting."

- Stress: A stimuli or situation that is perceived as threatening and leads to anxiety or other unpleasant emotions.

- Anxiety: An emotional reaction consisting of a combination of unpleasant:

  1) Thoughts and worries
  2) Feelings
  3) Physiological changes

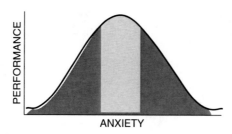

The Inverted-U Hypothesis

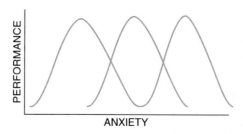

The Inverted-U Hypothesis and Sport Type

COGNITIVE KNOWLEDGE OF THE BODY IN SPORT PSYCHOLOGY

- Association

  - Directing attention to the sensations of effort and fatigue

    - Perceived exertion

    - Muscle tension

    - Pain and cramps

    - Respiration

    - Thirst

  - "I pay attention to my body."

  - "I read the signs."

  - "I have the equivalent of a shopping list that I keep going over."

  - "I tell myself to relax."

- Dissociation

  - Directing attention away from feelings of effort and fatigue

  - "The architect."

  - "The musician."

  - "The letter writer."

  - "The boss hater."

LUNG-GOM "SWIFTNESS OF FOOT"

- Practiced by Maheketang monks of Tibet

- Open gaze fixed on a distant object.

- Repeat a mantra in time with breathing.

- Link breathing with running pace.

POTENTIAL DANGERS OF DISSOCIATION

- Injury

- Overexertion

- Poor performance

THE STRESS OF TRAINING

- Staleness/Overtraining Syndrome

  - A long-term drop in performance due to intensive training training.

    - Depression and mood disturbances

    - Medical illness

    - Muscle soreness

    - Sleep disturbances

    - Loss of appetite

THE STRESS OF INACTIVITY

- At most, 22% of the U.S. population exercises 3 times a week for at least 20 minutes

- 24% of the U.S. population does not exercise at all

"The athlete, at work and at play constitutes a fine laboratory for the study of vexing physiological and psychological problems, many of which are distorted by the attempt to reduce them to simpler terms". (Coleman Roberts Griffith, 1925)

CHAPTER XVIII

YOUTH SPORT

Dr. Phil Henson
Department of Kinesiology
Indiana University

YOUTH SPORT

- 30 million children participate in youth sports

- _____ drop out by age 12

- 1 in 11,074 H.S. basketball players will make it to the NBA

- Less than 4000 professional athletes in the United States (.01%)

- Average pro career—_____ years

FORMER EAST GERMAN SYSTEM

- Some sports require early selection

  Gymnastics

  Swimming

- These same sports require tremendously long hours of practice and commitment.

- Are young kids ready to handle pressure of success?

- Most have overbearing coach, parent, or both.

PREADOLESCENT (JR. HIGH)

- Be concerned with the _____—not the _____.

- Understand and attempt to meet the needs of the child.

- Make athletic participation a _____ experience.

- Protect and support the child in situations he or she is not prepared to handle alone.

- Focus on small but meaningful goals, which are reinforced by appropriate rewards.

ADOLESCENT (HIGH SCHOOL)

- The coach must be a model of what he or she says.

- The coach must be willing to listen to and seriously consider the _____ of each athlete.

- The coach must never attempt to mislead or deceive the athlete.

- The coach must be prepared for periods of unusual _____.

- The coach must try to assume the role of a kind, considerate father or mother figure, rather than lord and master.

COLLEGE

- This is the first time that athletes may leave home and be placed in a situation because of their _____ in their sport.

- The athlete needs to have realistic goals based on his or her talent.

- The coach must be aware of _____ on the athlete.

- This is usually the first situation in which the _____ may have the opportunity to decide who will coach him or her.

- The athlete should begin preparing to make some of his or her own decisions about training, technique, etc.

CHAPTER XIX

MENTAL IMAGERY, REACTION TIME, AND PRACTICE SCHEDULES

Dr. Phil Henson
Department of Kinesiology
Indiana University

MENTAL IMAGERY

- Mental practice

- Mental rehearsal

- _____ —How detailed and realistic is the image?

- _____ —How can you make the image do what you want?

- Mental imagery prepares the motor pathways for the actual movement

  - Third person—seeing someone do something

  - Second person—seeing yourself do something

  - First person—feeling yourself do something (most effective)

- _____—gain in performance following rest.

- _____ practice results in greater performance improvement than physical practice alone or mental practice alone.

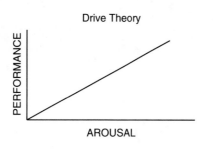

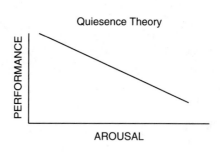

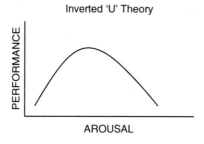

Performance Theories

REACTION TIME

- Stimulus picked up by a receptor

- Signal travels to _____ (afferent)

- Signal processed in brain

- Signal travels to _____ (efferent)

- Muscle initiates _____

FACTORS AFFECTING REACTION TIME

1. _____ (warning)

   - The period of time before the stimulus
   - 1-4 seconds is best

2. _____

   - Visual (slightly longer)
   - Auditory (strength of sound not so important)
   - Proprioceptive (linemen touching hands)
   - Pain is slower

3. Gender and Age

   - Males slightly faster
   - Optimal age 18-20; becomes slower with age past that

4. Simple vs. complex response

   - If decision is necessary, response is slower

5. Athletes have slightly faster reaction times

   - Which came first?

6. Practice

   - Improvement occurs with practice, to a point

LEARNING

- _____—performance gain in opposite limb

- **Practice** – Practice in a variety of situations similar to what is expected in competition

- _____—Better in learning simple task 1st time

- _____—Better in complex tasks; better in mental imagery

- **Audience**—_____ in learning new task; _____ in very complex task; _____ in simple task; _____ when skill is well-learned

- **Whole-Part-Whole**

  Part-Whole

  Technique--One or two things at a time

KNOWLEDGE OF RESULTS

- See result

- Hear about result

- Know result

- Example: basketball free throw

- _____—decrease in motor performance during practice

REACTION TIME

- *Sensory nerve—*_____

- *Motor nerve—*_____

- *Reaction time*—the time between stimulus and voluntary muscle movement

- *Components*

  - Pre motor

  - Motor time—the time between muscle firing and movement

- *Movement time*

  - Force involved (resistance)

  - Strength of stimulus

  - Muscle tension

- _____—nerve and muscle fibers it activates (all or none)

- *Speed of reaction*

  - _____ fibers faster

  - _____ fibers are faster

  - _____ fiber is slower

  - _____ occur at spinal cord level

CHAPTER XX

FITNESS AND HEALTH

Dr. Jeanne D. Johnston
Department of Kinesiology
Indiana University

RESEARCH

- Interpret popular media and advertisements
- Understand how protocol is decided
  - The "why' of exercise
- Understand physiological principles
- Recognize differences in populations

CAUSES OF HUMAN DISEASE

- Lifestyle

  – _____

  – _____ Smoking, diet, stress, physical activity
- Genetics

OBESITY

- _____: Having a very high amount of body fat in relation to lean body mass

- _____: A measure of an adult's weight in relation to height (kg/height (m)^2)

BMI CLASSIFICATIONS

- Acceptable range 20 – 25

- Overweight (BMI 25.1 – 29.9)

- Obese (BMI 30>)

- Morbidly obese (BMI > 40.0)

CURRENT STATUS OF OBESITY

- _____ Adult U.S. population overweight or obese

  - ~33% obese, ~5% morbidly obese

- Percentages are increasing: 15.0% (1976) to 32.9% (2004)

- Children

  - 2–5 yrs: 5.0% to 13.9%

  - 6–11 yrs: 5% to 18.8%

  - 12–19 yrs: 5.0% to 17.4%.

- Estimate _____ of Americans will be overweight or obese by 2015

WHAT ARE WE DOING AS A NATION?

- Healthy People 2010 Goal: 15%

- National strategy to combat obesity

- Indiana Health Weight Initiative

  - InShape Indiana

COST OF OBESITY

- GDP 8.8% (1980) to 17.6% (2009)

- What does that mean as an individual?

WHAT CAN YOU DO?

- Knowledgeable ambassador
  - Education
  - Experience
- Enthusiasm
- Proactive
- Lead by example

REDUCTION IN PHYSICAL ACTIVITY REQUIRED IN DAILY LIFE

- EE required to sustain food supply
- Safe and rapid _____
- _____ in work
- Changes in _____
- Change in _____

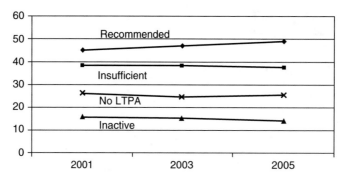

Reported Physical Activity by Adults in the USA: 2001–2005 Data from BRFSS

- Recommended: _____

- Insufficient: >10 min/wk MOD or VPA but less than recommended

- Inactive: <10 min/wk lifestyle activities

- No LTPA

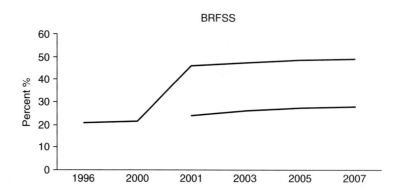

ALL PA:

  1996 – 2000: 30 min any PA 5 or > days/week

  2001 – 2007: 30 min MPA 5 or > days/wk OR VPA 20 min, 3> days/wk

VIG PA: 20+ min 3 or more days/week

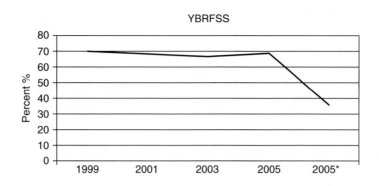

1999 – 2005: 20 min VPA 3 days/wk or 30 min MPA 5 days/wk

New 2005: 60 min MOD or VIG 5 or > days/wk

SECTORS OF HEALTH/FITNESS INDUSTRY

- Corporate

- Community

- Commercial

- Clinical

WHY WORKSITE WELLNESS?

- More than 60% of adults work, and many spend 2,000 or more hours a year at work.

  - 123 million adults aged 20 – 64

  - 55% men, 11% African American, 15% Hispanic

  - 51% aged 40-64

- Worksite wellness makes the places they work healthier.

- An ideal healthy worksite has opportunities for employees to:

  - be physically active

  - eat healthful foods

  - live tobacco-free

CORPORATE VIEW

- Rising healthcare costs

- Ford spent _____ for healthcare of 550,000 employees and retirees (2006).

- General Motors spent _____ for healthcare of 1.1 million employees

- Reduce costs

  - Federal tax cut?

WHY CORPORATE FITNESS

- _____ absenteeism

- _____ productivity

- _____ injuries

- _____ medical costs

- _____ morale

- Employee recruitment

- Employee retention

- Healthy Workplace 2010

ACTIVITIES

- Health fairs

- Health screening services

- Health promotion seminars

- Behavior change programs

- Weight management

- Fitness and health promotion programming

- Group exercise classes

- Membership recruitment and retention

- Fitness testing and evaluation

- Recreation programming

WORKSITE WELLNESS PROGRAMS

- Strengths
  - Health risk appraisals
  - Health screenings
  - Education
- Weaknesses
  - One size fits all attitude
  - Lack of diversity in interventions
  - Change environment
  - Change behavior

COMMUNITY

- Organizations: YMCA
- Hotels
- Hospitals
- University
- Local and state
  - Recreation programs
  - Communities designed for activity
  - INShape Indiana

COMMERCIAL

- For-profit business

- Single purpose: Gold's gym

- Multipurpose: Racquet club

- Franchise: Bally Total Fitness

- Health clubs

- Fitness equipment

- Supplements

CLINICAL

- Cardiac and pulmonary rehabilitation

- Cancer rehabilitation

- Diabetes clinics: education and care

- Sports medicine

- Physical therapy

- Pharmaceutical companies

WHAT IS YOUR ROLE?

- _____
- _____
- _____
- _____

INDIANA UNIVERSITY RESEARCH PROJECTS

- Physical Activity, health, wellness, and quality of life

  – Worksite, college, master athletes

  – Technology, games

  – Obesity Index

- Asthma

- Performance based:

  – Milk!!!

  – Recovery

  – Swimming

- Cardiovascular disease

  – Hypertension: Short bouts

  – Post-meal lipid profile

CHAPTER XXI

EXERCISE AND DISEASE: PREVENTION AND TREATMENT OF CANCER, HEART DISEASE, OBESITY, AND DIABETES

Shayla Holtkamp, BS Kinesiology, MPH
Department of Applied Health Science
Indiana University

CANCER

Most common cancers

- Men

  – _____

  – Lung

  – Colorectal

  – Stomach (Asian/Pacific Island), Bladder (white men), mouth and throat (black men)

- Women

  – _____

  – Lung

  – Colorectal

  – Uterine (endometrial)

PHYSICAL ACTIVITY AND CANCER

- Convincing evidence that physical activity is associated with reduced risk for

    - Colon cancer

    - Breast cancer

- Several studies have reported links between physical activity and reduced risk of cancers of

    - Prostate

    - Lung

    - Endometrium

BREAST CANCER

- Physical activity reduces risk by _____

- Both pre-menopausal and post

- Greatest benefits were among women of normal weight

    - Not found in obese and overweight

- Change in hormone balance, body mass, and immune function preventing tumor development

PROSTATE CANCER

- Physical activity reduces risk for cancer by _____

- Small number of studies suggest inactive men have higher rate compared to very active men

- Biological mechanisms are unknown

COLON CANCER

- Physical activity reduces risk by _____

- Physical activity aids in regular bowel movements, decreasing exposure to carcinogens

- Causes changes in metabolism and hormone levels reducing tumor development

- Alters number of inflammatory and immune factors

EXERCISE AND CANCER-RELATED FATIGUE

- Newer research

  - Exercise is not only safe but can improve physical functioning and quality of life

- Benefits to cancer patient:

  - Better blood flow to legs

  - Less dependence on others

  - Improved self-esteem

  - Lower anxiety and depression

  - Less nausea

  - *Fewer symptoms of fatigue*

CANCER-RELATED FATIGUE

Meta-analysis of 28 studies:

- Exercise is more effective at combating the problem than the usual care provided: Told to expect fatigue and accept it

- Studies:

  - 12-week intervention

  - Walking 30 minutes per day 3-5 days per week

EXERCISE SAFETY AND PRECAUTIONS FOR CANCER SURVIVORS

Always check with doctor. Don't exercise if:

- You are _____

- You have low white blood cell counts (stay away from public places!)

- You mineral levels are not normal

- You are overly _____

- You have bleeding if you are taking blood thinners

- You have unrelieved pain, nausea/vomiting

- Don't expose skin that has had radiation to the chlorine in swimming pools

CORONARY HEART DISEASE

- _____ single killer of American males and females

- 2009 estimated direct and indirect cost of CHD is $165.4 billion

HEART DISEASE

RISK FACTORS

- Physical in-activity
- High blood pressure
- High cholesterol
- Diabetes
- Stress
- Smoking
- Obesity

MORE RISK FACTORS

- Those that can't be changed
  - Increasing age
  - Gender
  - Heredity

EXERCISE AND PREVENTION AND TREATMENT OF HEART DISEASE

- Primary prevention

  Actions taken to avoid disease or injury.

- Secondary prevention

  Actions taken to identify and treat an illness or injury early on with the aim of stopping or reversing the problem

- Tertiary prevention

  Interventions to contain or retard the damage caused by a serious injury or a disease that has progressed beyond the early stages and causes lasting or irreversible damage

PRIMARY PREVENTION

- Exercise

- Eat healthy

- Don't smoke

- Maintain a desirable body weight

- Could account for an 84% reduction of risk

SECONDARY PREVENTION

- Identify those at high risk for disease

  - Screening

  - Taking blood pressure, etc.

- Identify those with disease

- Treat and rehabilitate those with disease

- Secondary prevention can:

  - Decrease need for interventional procedures (angioplasty)

  - Reduce incidence of another heart attack

TERTIARY PREVENTION

- Treatment after a coronary event

  - _____

  - _____

  - _____

- _____

- Preventing further deterioration and increasing quality of life

PREVENTION AND TREATMENT OF OBESITY

- Lack of "energy balance"

- Genetics

- Amount of physical activity to prevent unhealthy weight gain will vary from individual to individual

- _____ will increase the likelihood of success

EXERCISE AND OBESITY

- Exercise might be even more important for weight management

- Importance of strength training

- Need more than 3–5 days per week

- Lifestyle activities

EXERCISE AND TYPE 2 DIABETES

- "Diabetes Prevention Program (DPP) study conclusively showed that people with pre-diabetes can prevent the development of type 2 diabetes by making changes in diet and increasing their level of exercise."

    – May be able to return blood glucose levels to normal range

    – DDP also showed that some medications may delay development BUT exercise worked better

TREATMENT OF TYPE 2 DIABETES

- Endurance activities and strength training is an underutilized therapeutic modality

- _____ is imperative to sustain glucose-lowering effect and improved insulin sensitivity

WHAT TYPES OF EXERCISE?

- _____

  - Study: 16 weeks of strength training produced dramatic improvements in sugar control comparable to diabetes medication

- _____

  - Decreases risk of type 2 diabetes
  - Helps to manage blood sugar levels

CHAPTER XXII

ATHLETIC TRAINING: EDUCATIONAL PREPARATION AND CURRENT CONCEPTS OF PRACTICE

Dr. Katie Grove, LAT, ATC
Dr. Joanne Klossner, LAT, ATC
Dr. Carrie Docherty-Steele, LAT, ATC
Department of Kinesiology
Indiana University

ATHLETIC TRAINING

- What is AT?

- Undergraduate program

- Graduate program

- Job opportunities

- Injuries

WHAT IS ATHLETIC TRAINING?

Six Domains of athletic Training

- _____ of athletic injuries

- Clinical _____ and diagnosis

- _____ care of injuries

- _____, rehabilitation, and reconditioning

- Organization and administration

- Professional responsibilities

FACTS ABOUT ATHLETIC TRAINERS

- Athletic trainers are recognized as allied healthcare professionals

- An independent national board certifies athletic trainers

- _____ of athletic trainers have a master's or doctoral degree

- More than _____ of athletic trainers work outside the traditional school setting

- 30,000+ members of the Athletic Training profession (NATA)

INDIANA UNIVERSITY

One of the few programs that has both an undergraduate and graduate program

- BS Athletic Training

- MS Kinesiology, Emphasis in Athletic Training

INDIANA UNIVERSITY – UNDERGRADUATE ATEP OVERVIEW

- Admission criteria

- Curriculum

- Clinical assignment

- Job placement

ADMISSION CRITERIA

- Applications due April 1

- Criteria for admission to the Athletic Training Program are:

    — Application

    — Interview

    — Completion of HPER H160 and HPER P280 with a B or higher

    — Completion of ANAT A215, Human Anatomy, with a C or higher

    — University GPA of 2.5 or higher

    — Complete Technical Standards /signed by physician

    — Observation – 12 hours (assigned through P280)

ADMISSION SELECTION

Selection is based on

- GPA and grades in the three required courses (35%)

- Letters of recommendation (20%)

- Interview (45%)

- Please note:
  This major is intended to prepare athletic trainers and is not intended as a stepping stone to other allied health professions. Students applying who plan to be athletic trainers will be given the **HIGHEST priority**.

APPLICATION

http://www.indiana.edu/~kines/undergraduate/training.shtml

CURRICULUM

Three-Year Program

- Assessment of Athletic Injuries, Strapping & Bandaging, General Medical, Therapeutic Modalities, Clinical Education

- Therapeutic Rehabilitation, Clinical Education

- Senior Seminar, Organization and Administration, Clinical Education

JOB OPPORTUNITIES

- Clinics

- High Schools

- College/ University

- Professional

- Industrial

- Special Settings

ATHLETIC TRAINERS IN SPECIAL SETTINGS

http://www.nata.org/about_AT/worksettings.htm

A DAY IN THE LIFE OF A COLLEGIATE ATHLETIC TRAINER . . . .

Basic Day in the Life:

- 7:00 am   @ work: treatments

- 9:00–10:00   Teach class

- 10:00–noon   Treatment

- 1:00–3:00   Pre-practice

- 3:00–5:30   Practice

- 5:30–7:00   Post-practice treatment

Add in weekend competitions and travel time.

QUESTIONS

Dr. Katie Grove, LAT, ATC
Director, Athletic Training Education
kagrove@indiana.edu

Dr. Joanne Klossner, LAT, ATC
Clinical Coordinator, Athletic Training Education
jklossne@indiana.edu

CHAPTER XXIII

PHYSICAL THERAPY

Cindy Moore
Coordinator of Academic Advising
Department of Kinesiology
Indiana University

WHAT IS PHYSICAL THERAPY?

- Healthcare profession that provides treatment and services to individuals to develop and maintain and restore movement and function and promote overall fitness and health.

  – Circumstances leading to the necessity of treatment are:

    - Aging

    - Injury

    - Disease

    - Environmental factors

- Physical therapists work with patients in a variety of settings:

  – Hospitals

  – Outpatient clinics

  – Private practices

  – Sport and fitness facilities

  – Home healthcare agencies

  – Nursing homes

  – Work settings

- Physical therapists help patients with a variety of physical disabilities and diseases:

  – Low-back pain

  – Arthritis

  – Heart disease

  – Fractures

  – Head injuries

  – Cerebral palsy

EMPLOYMENT FACTS FOR PHYSICAL THERAPISTS

- In 2008 – Physical Therapists held about 185,00 jobs in the United States (U.S. Bureau of Labor Statistics)

- In 2008 – Median annual salary $72,790. (U.S. Bureau of Labor Statistics)

- In 2008 – Job outlook for physical therapists is projected to be excellent; occupation is projected to experience fast growth through 2018. (U.S. Bureau of Labor Statistics)

EDUCATIONAL REQUIREMENTS FOR PHYSICAL THERAPY

- Students wanting to practice physical therapy in the United States must now have a DPT degree – Doctorate in Physical Therapy

  - Bachelor's degree from an accredited 4-year undergraduate program is required for admission to a DPT program

- DPT programs are 3-year programs that include both class work and practical work

- Undergraduate requirements:

  - Most programs require a bachelor's degree from an accredited institution

  - Prerequisite course work for most schools include:

    - General Chemistry – 2 semesters (4-5 cr.) – each must include a lab

    - General Physics – 2 semesters (4-5 cr.) – each must include a lab

    - Human Anatomy – 1 semester (4-5 cr.) – must include a lab

    - Human Physiology – 1 semester (4-5 cr.) – must include a lab

    - Biology – 1 or 2 semesters (4 cr.) – including lab (depends on the school)

    - English Composition

    - General Psychology

    - Statistics

    - Mathematics – generally college algebra or higher

    - Life Span Development or Developmental Psychology

    - Medical Terminology

    - Additional social sciences

    - Possible additional humanities (including Ethics)

    - Shadowing hours (number of hours varies – see each school's requirements)

- Most programs also require students to take the GRE – Graduate Record Examination – required for entrance to most graduate programs

LICENSURE

- All states regulate the practice of physical therapy

  – Eligibility varies by state

- Typical requirements:

  – Graduate from accredited PT program

  – Pass the National Physical Therapy Examination

  – Fulfill state requirements, such as state licensing exams

  – Most states will require Continuing Education as a condition of maintaining licensure

ADVANCEMENT IN THE PT FIELD

- PTs are expected to continue professional development

  – Continuing Education Courses

  – Workshops

- Some become Board Certified in a clinical specialty

- Some PTs go into academia and research

- Some become self-employed

  – Contract services

  – Open private practice

CHAPTER XXIV

CAREERS IN KINESIOLOGY: ACADEMIC AND CAREER ADVISING

Dr. Susan Simmons

Cindy Moore
Department of Kinesiology
Indiana University

MAJORS AND CAREERS IN KINESIOLOGY

The majors in the Department of Kinesiology are professional degrees. They prepare you to go out into the work world into entry level positions.

ACADEMIC ADVISING SERVICES

- Provide information needed for academic planning

  - Assist you with degree progress and academic policies using your academic advising report

- Explain academic policies

- Refer students to other sources of help

  - Referrals to other academic units or student assistance centers – Counseling & Psychological Services (CAPS), Student Academic Centers (SAC), Disabled Student Services (DSS), Student Advocates

- Direct students to resources that can be used for employment and grad school planning

KINESIOLOGY CAREER SERVICES

Susan E. C. Simmons, Ph.D.

- Director of Career Placement

- Assists students with finding internships and jobs

- Assists students in setting up internships and practicum experiences

- Will help students by reviewing resumes and cover letters that are going to potential employers

- Will help students writing personal statements for graduate school

- Will help students prepare for jobs/grad school by conducting mock interviews

- Runs the HPER Careers website – www.HPERcareers.com

SEVEN ACADEMIC MAJORS IN THE DEPARTMENT OF KINESIOLOGY

1. Physical Education

   - K-12 Teaching

   - Health

   - Coaching

   - Athletic Training – this is actually a second degree and will take 5 years to complete

2. Exercise (Sport) Science

   - Professional schools:

     – Medicine

     – Physical Therapy

     – Physician's Assistant

     – Occupational Therapist

     – Optometry

     – Other medical specialties:

       - Sports Medicine

       - Cardiopulmonary Rehabilitation Specialist

   - Graduate schools:

     – Exercise Physiology

     – Preventive/Rehabilitative Exercise

     – Biomechanics

     – Motor Learning

     – Psychology of Sport

     – Sociology of Sport

3. Fitness Specialist

- Fitness clubs
- Personal training
- Group exercise leader
- Strength and conditioning
- Fitness management

4. Athletic Training

- High school
- College
- Professional
- Clinics
- Industrial

5. Sports Marketing and Management

- Athletic administration
- Sales and promotions
- Community relations
- Operations/Facility management
- Governing bodies
    - USOC
    - NGBs
    - City Sports Corp.
- Sports agencies
- Professional schools (MBA/Law)

6. Sports Communication (Broadcast and Print)

   - Journalism (Print)
   - Radio/Television (Broadcast)
   - Sports information (media)
   - Public relations
   - Photojournalism

7. Dance

   - Performance
   - Choreography
   - Pedagogy
   - Yoga/Pilates

THE BIG QUESTIONS!

- What do I want to do when I finish school?
- What can I do with a degree in Kinesiology?

There are lots of choices!

CHOICE IS GOOD!

But choice also makes the decision-making process more difficult.

HOW CAN THE CAREER CENTER HELP?

Resources and Services to unlock your career potential:

- Resumes and cover letters

- Internships

- Job search

- Interview skills

- Career counseling

SO HOW DO I CHOOSE A CAREER PATH?

- Determine your interests

- Assess your strengths and weaknesses

- Think about the workplace setting

- Consider work/life balance (hours and responsibilities)

- Evaluate your salary requirements

- Analyze your career goals and opportunities for advancement

- Try it out . . . gain experience

- *Getting started with an action plan*

DEVELOP A CAREER ACTION PLAN

Four Steps

- Discovery

- Exploration

- Experience and Experiment

- Choice

INTERNSHIPS: WHY ARE THEY IMPORTANT?

- Explore and clarify major and career goals

- Develop related- knowledge, competencies, and experience

- Gain practical experience that will be desirable to employers

- Rewarding – puts learning in your hands

- Establish a network of contacts, mentors, and references

INTERNSHIPS – WHAT ARE MY OPTIONS?

- Personal training

- Group exercise

- Nonprofit organizations (such as YMCA)

- Performance training

- Corporate fitness

- Commercial fitness

- Fitness spa/ranch

- Recreational fitness/collegiate setting

- Heath/wellness education

- Cardiac rehabilitation

- Physical therapy

RECEIVING COURSE CREDIT FOR AN INTERNSHIP

- Meet with career counselor if you need help finding an internship

- Locate and land the internship

- Complete an internship agreement form and return it to career center for authorization

- Register for credit

- Complete internship hours

- Complete final evaluations

- Complete exit interview

CHAPTER XXV

OLYMPIC SPORTS

Dr. Phil Henson
Department of Kinesiology
Indiana University

OLYMPICS

HISTORY

- Ancient Olympic Games
- Modern Olympic Games (1896)
- Leisure class
- Working class

USOC – UNITED STATES OLYMPIC COMMITTEE

- Annual budget--$85 million

- $20 million to NGBs

- $8.5 million to athletes support

ATLANTA – SUMMER GAMES 1996

- 1.7 billion

- 540 million sponsors

- 555 million TV viewers

- 600 million tickets and Miscellaneous includes clothing, souveniors, etc.

FUND RAISING

- Future fund raising is likely to suffer

- Dream team

- Soviet Union breakup

- **Ideas**

  - Reduce nationalism

  - Eliminate team sports

  - Eliminate subjective judging

  - Hold Olympics in multiple locations

OLYMPIC SPORTS

- Objective (timed or measured)

- Subjective (judged)

- Combative

- Team

EXAM 1 STUDY GUIDE

The following are terms and concepts you should know, understand, and be able to apply. You are also responsible for anything else in the lecture notes or textbook chapters.

% oxygen in the air

Acclimatization

Acid-base balance

ADP

Aerobic

Alveoli

Anabolic

Anaerobic

Aorta

Arteries

ATP

Body composition

Breathe Rite

Bronchial tubes

Carbohydrate

Carbon dioxide

Cardiac output

Catabolic

Diastole

Diffusion

Disciplines in Exercise Science

Energy

Energy systems

Environment

Factors not represented by MAX VO_2

Factors that stimulate respiration (breathing)

Fat

Female Triad

Fitness

Genetics

Heart rate

Hematocrit

Hemoglobin

Hypothesis

Lactic acid

Lung Size

MAX VO_2

Metabolism

Negative pressure breathing

Nitrogen

Null hypothesis

Oxidation

Oxygen

Pulmonic circulation

Photosynthesis

Protein

Respiratory quotient

Scientific method

Starling's law

Stroke volume

Systemic circulation

Systole

Trachea

Veins

Work

EXAM 2 STUDY GUIDE

The following are terms and concepts you should know, understand, and be able to apply. You are also responsible for anything else in the lecture notes or textbook chapters.

Acceleration

Adrenalin

Aggression

Altitude

Amenorrhea

Anabolic steroids

Anaerobic threshold

Anorexia

Arteriosclerosis

ATP & ADP

Barometric pressure

Biomechanics

Blood boosting and blood doping

Body fat

Bulimia

Calcium retention

Carbohydrate

Carbon dioxide

Center of gravity

Curvilinear motion

Eating disorder

Eccentric thrust

Ergogenic aid

Estrogen

Fat

Fatigue

Female Triad

Fitness

Frostbite

Half the barometric pressure

Heat balance

Hemoglobin

Hydration

Hormone

Hypobaric hypoxia

Hypertrophy

Hyperplasia

Instinct

Lean body mass

Linear motion

Mitochondria

Moment of inertia

Newton's laws of motion

Nitrogen

Osteoporosis

Oxygen

Parabola

Placebo

Protein

Rehabilitation

RICE

Rotary motion

Testosterone

Transfer of momentum

Title IX

Velocity

FINAL EXAM STUDY GUIDE

The following are terms and concepts you should know, understand, and be able to apply. You are also responsible for anything else in the lecture notes or textbook chapters.

Great athletes/coaching

Types of coaches (leaders)

Sport injuries

RICE

Physical therapist

Athletic trainer

Motor learning

Motor control

Skill

Ability

Drive theory

Quiescence theory

IZOF

Inverted-U theory

Massed practice

Distributed practice

Mental imagery

Reaction time

Knowledge of results

Knowledge of performance

Play

Games

Sport

Golden Age of Sport

Graduation ratios of athletes/non-athletes

Sport psychology

Domains of learning

Reminiscence

Henneman's size principle

Neural plasticity

Title IX

Conflict theory

Functionalist theory

Critical theory

Youth sports

ADDENDUM I — 80 YEARS OF BASKETBALL — A PERSONAL REFLECTION

Dr. John M. Cooper
Professor Emeritus
Indiana University

JOHN M. COOPER — ONE OF THE ORIGINATORS OF THE JUMP SHOT

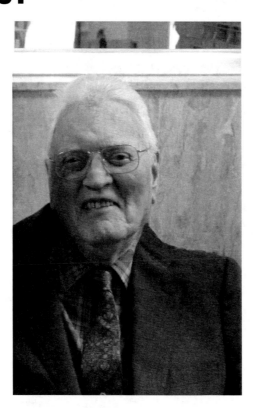

STATE OF MISSOURI BASKETBALL HALL OF FAME SPRINGFIELD, MISSOURI

- In the 1920s a young boy playing high school basketball found himself with a small problem. John Cooper constantly looked up to everyone else on the court. "All the fellas on the team were bigger and older than I was," Cooper said. "They would slap the ball down every time I would throw it up in practice."

JOHN M. COOPER

- Cooper's solution: the jump shot. "I would just jump up and shoot it in the air before I came down to get it over them." The jump shot was a radical idea. Until that time the accepted form of outside shooting was the two-handed set shot. Cooper scored over 500 points in one season in high school, an amount unheard of in those days.

- Cooper went on to attend the University of Missouri, where he played for the Tigers from 1930–34. Playing for Mizzou, Cooper took his jump shot on the road. He is the first player to use the shot as a primary offensive weapon. "The defenses kept catching up with the offense, so the offense had to do something else." In the '31–'32 season Cooper accounted for 47% of Missouri's scoring. It was not the shot heard around the world, but it did mark the start of an evolution of the game if not a revolution in the game.

JOHN M. COOPER'S BASKETBALL EXPERIENCE

- Started playing on the high school team in the 8th grade.

- Played as a starter in high school from freshman year on.

- As a player at the University of Missouri, tied for individual scoring championship in conference.

- Coached in high school for 6 years, 1934–40.

- After college, played on several teams, 1934–1940, known as AAU or town teams.

- Served as assistant coach at the University of Missouri, 1940–42.

- Selected to play in St. Louis on a team playing against a regular traveling AAU team for Finnish Relief; voted co-MVP of the game.

- Served as captain of an undefeated Air Force team during World War II.

- Coached AAU team in Los Angeles just after World War II.

  – Tea'm finished 4th in Nationals at Oklahoma City.

- Played basketball on a team until 52 years of age.

- Provided scouting reports of certain games as requested.

- Authored two books on basketball.

- Researched performances of players.

- Studied films of players and gave reports of action.

- Taught basketball classes at the University of Southern California for twenty years.

- Gave demonstrations at several colleges on how basketball was played 60 years ago.

ONE HUNDRED YEARS OF RULES – A SELECTION OF KEY RULES

- 1911 – 4 foul limit for players; no coaching allowed during progress of the game.

- 1924 – Player fouled must shoot own free throws; previously one player usually shot all of them for the team.

- 1933 – 10-second line added as anti-stall device. <u>3-second rule (in lane) introduced, only for player with ball.</u>

- 1936 – Center jump eliminated after free throws were made; team scored against awarded out-ofbounds possession.

  – 3-second rule applied to all players.

- 1938 – Center jump eliminated after field goals, too.

- 1943 – Players still in game at start of overtime permitted to play until fifth foul.

- 1949 – Coaches permitted to talk to teams during time-out.

JOHN M. COOPER – PERSONAL EXPERIENCES

- Played against a coal mining team in high school; results were amazing.

- Played on a basketball court with one side against a stage.

- Played against a left-handed player.

- In a game against Kansas State, I faked a shot, drove for the basket, then fell into a lady's lap. "Oh my!"

- When the ball rolled around the rim on a shot bya teammate, I jumped up to tip it in and got hung up on the net next to the rim of the basket.

- If a shooter was successful when he shot, he was off to the races, but if he was not successful on the first or second shot, he had a bad shooting game. This was known by his opponents.

- On a lay up, I cracked into the iron support back of the goal.
  A physician had to sew up my mouth.

- Adjusted to a court with only one side open. The other side was against the wall.

- An Oklahoma player did some hazing by calling me "pretty boy."
  I was bothered by this. Only women and girls are pretty.

- The team went to UCLA for a practice game. The court surface was slick.

- Usually top players have height, big hands,thin lower legs, and quick feet. Some have great height and use that to move lighter players.

- Many high school teams from small high schools in my vicinity played the game on outdoor courts. We often wore caps to shade against the sun. You had to learn to catch the cap if it started to fall. You did this while on the move.

- One team used the tactic of having a player step forward and say, "Let me throw the ballin." He would pass to his teammate and score a basket.

- When near the basket, a USC player faked a shot with the ball between the legs. We had never seen this done. Our Missouri team was upset in that game.

- In a game against Kansas, our coach decided that we should get an early lead and stall by sitting on the ball. We did this until the end of the first half. We started the second half the same way (holding the ball). Kansas had enough and came with a rush. We were able to hold them off and won. This was the origin of the
  10 second rule.

- Kansas had enough of a small post man, which I was, and succeeded in getting the 3 second rule passed. There also was support for this from other sources.

- When I was in high school, we played in the state tournament against a team that used a bounce pass. We did not know what to do and lost the game in the quarter finals.